VIRUSES,

PLAGUES,

AND

HISTORY

MICHAEL B. A. OLDSTONE

OXFORD

UNIVERSITY PRESS

OXFORD
UNIVERSITY PRESS

Oxford   New York

Athens   Auckland   Bangkok   Bogotá   Buenos Aires
Calcutta   Cape Town   Chennai   Dar es Salaam   Delhi
Florence   Hong Kong   Istanbul   Karachi
Kuala Lumpur   Madrid   Melbourne   Mexico City
Mumbai   Nairobi   Paris   São Paulo   Singapore
Taipei   Tokyo   Toronto   Warsaw

and associated companies in
Berlin   Ibadan

First Published by Oxford University Press, Inc., 1998
198 Madison Avenue, New York, New York 10016

First issued as an Oxford University Press Paperback, 2000

Oxford is a registered trademark of Oxford University Press

Library of Congress Cataloging-in-Publication Data
Oldstone, Michael B. A.
Viruses, plagues, and history / by Michael B. A. Oldstone
p.   cm.   Includes bibliographical references and index.
ISBN 0-19-511723-9 (Cloth)
ISBN 0-19-513422-2 (Pbk.)
1. Virus diseases—History. I. Title
RC114.5.037   1998
614.5'7—dc21 8 97-9545

1 3 5 7 9 10 8 6 4 2
Printed in the United States of America

VIRUSES,

PLAGUES,

AND

HISTORY

FOR BETSY,
JENNY, BEAU, AND CHRIS

CONTENTS

PREFACE

This book was conceived in the spirit of Paul deKruif's book *Microbe Hunters*, which I first read in junior high school. His heroes were the great adventurers of medical science who engaged in a struggle to understand the unknown and relieve human suffering. In retrospect, those stories initiated the spark that led me to medical school and a career in biomedical research. From those opportunities, I came to know Hilary Koprowski, Jonas Salk, Albert Sabin, Tom Weller, Bob Gallo, Luc Montagnier, D. A. Henderson, Jordie Casals, Rob Webster, D. Carlton Gajdusek, Joe Gibbs, Stanley Prusiner, and Bruce Chesebro, all of whom figure in the stories told here about viral diseases.

In tracing the history of struggles to find each agent of these diseases, I have asked what was known from its initial description, what unique problems existed, what actions were the most critical in solving the problems, why these decisions were made, and at what point community and governmental support provided the essential resources. To accomplish this task, I selected as examples four viral diseases—smallpox, yellow fever, measles, and poliomyelitis—that science has harnessed despite the unrestrained devastation and misery they once caused. These success stories are contrasted with those of four viral infections that remain out of control—Lassa fever virus, Ebola virus, Hantavirus, and human immunodeficiency virus—and with the continuing threat from influenza, now reasonably contained but with the potential to revert to a worldwide pandemic disaster. I also tell the story of an unusual group of progressive neurologic disorders, the spongiform encephalopathies (scrapie, mad cow disease, Creutzfeldt–Jakob disease), and the debate as to whether they are caused by a virus or a prion (protein). A common thread of fear, superstition, and irrational behavior runs through all ten stories, testifying to our human fallibility. However, the motivation and skill of scientists along with the right community and governmental support have led to important victories over some viral plagues, and there will be more.

This book commemorates the enormous magnitude of these achievements, perhaps too often forgotten. Recall that smallpox killed over 300 million people in the twentieth century alone and now has been eradicated. Measles, which once killed millions each year globally and still does so in

Third World countries, today harms few in the industrial countries of the world. Yellow fever virus devastated populations along the Mississippi River and several port cities in the United States and was responsible for closing operations of the American government in 1793. Now this infectious disease has been eradicated from the United States, although it still exists in rain forests of South America and Africa. Poliomyelitis virus, the cause of infantile paralysis, was at one time the fifth leading killer of children in Scandinavia and pervasive in North America. I remember my parents' fear of poliomyelitis each summer, a fear that is still vivid in the minds of many of us over forty years of age who saw siblings, schoolmates or friends stricken, then either die or become crippled. Yet once the American people and government as well as other governments invested in basic scientific research, poliomyelitis was brought under control, so that in neither Scandinavia nor the Americas is there a case of wild-type poliomyelitis today.

The most important benefit of controlling infectious diseases is alleviation of pain and suffering. Also a substantial benefit is the monetary saving, funds no longer required for hospitalization and treatment. Individuals who would otherwise have been incapacitated are now healthy, able to work, buy goods, and pay taxes. A safe estimate is that for each dollar invested by the government in basic research to study these diseases, a return of at least 1000-fold has been realized in terms of those who are financially productive, instead of requiring long-term care. Yet with success comes complacency, and a lessening of general awareness that viral diseases will always remain a threat. Only with continuing research can humankind hope to control those diseases that remain or are newly discovered and prevent the reemergence of viruses that were once tamed.

This book is based largely on the personal reports, letters, and messages of the principal persons involved. I have tried as far as possible to write from the original sources and from contemporary accounts by participants who saw the events firsthand as they unfolded. I have been fortunate to have the opportunity to become friends with many of those who played commanding roles in the fight to control and eradicate the viruses and to discuss with them many episodes described in this book. At medical school, I came under the influence of Theodore Woodward, a superb teacher and clinician who, as Chairman of Medicine at the University of Maryland, educated me in clinical aspects of infectious diseases. Through his urging and that of Charles Wisseman, Chair of the Microbiology Department, I was sent one summer to work at Walter Reed Hospital and Institute of Research. There I came in direct contact with Joseph Smadel, a dean of the scientific discipline of virology. Soon afterward I met John Enders, who recommended that, upon completion of the medical program, I apply my training in infectious diseases to the newly emerging field of immunology. Both Enders and Smadel play prominent roles in this book. Following Enders's advice, I moved to La Jolla to train under Frank Dixon, one of the major figures of immunology, at the Scripps Clinic and Research Foundation (now the Scripps Research Institute). The late 1960s and early '70s brought the opportunity to complement my immunologic training under Dixon and receive virologic training by working with virologist Karl Habel.

I am especially grateful to Hilary Koprowski, Jonas Salk, Albert Sabin, Tom Weller, Samuel Katz, D. A. Henderson, Frank Fenner, John Skehel, Brian Mahy, Jordie Casals, Luc Montagnier, and Robert Gallo as contributors to this history. Of course, I have consulted the voluminous literature on the subject, and I am indebted to Paula King and Marisela Perez-Meza of the Scripps Research Institute Medical Library for their assistance. I am also indebted to Brian Mahy and C. J. Peters, both personal friends and senior virologists at the Centers for Disease Control, Atlanta, Georgia, for their discussions on Lassa fever, Ebola virus, and Hantavirus infections.

I am particularly indebted to the Rockefeller Foundation, which provided me with a scholarship to live at the Villa Serbelloni, Bellagio, Italy, a sanctuary where I put many of my thoughts into words and constructed the outline for this book. Throughout the project I was fortunate to have the assistance of Gay Schilling, who provided expert secretarial services, and Phyllis Minick, who gave editorial advice, as well as my scientific colleagues; Frank J. Dixon, J. Lindsay Whitton, and Curtis Wilson (The Scripps Research Institute, La Jolla), Thomas Merigan (Stanford Medical School, Palo Alto), John Skehel (Medical Research Council, Mill Hill, London), Rob Webster (St. Jude Children's Research Hospital, Memphis), Bruce Chesebro (Rocky Mountain Laboratory, National Institutes of Health, Hamilton, Montana), and Sven Gard and Erling Norrby (Karolinska Institute, Stockholm), who offered valuable suggestions and comments on several of the chapters. I thank Kirk Jensen, editor at Oxford University Press, for his encouragement, advice, and faith in this book from its very beginning.

La Jolla, California   M.B.A.O.
Spring 1997

PART ONE

VIRUSES

PLAGUES,

AND HISTORY

You need not fear the terror by night,
nor the arrow that flies by day,
nor the plague that stalks in the darkness.

—91st Psalm

CHAPTER 1

A GENERAL
INTRODUCTION

Individual viruses have evolved interesting and unique lifestyles. One consequence is that battles have been won or lost when a particular virus infected one army but not its adversaries. Viruses have depleted the native populations of several continents. Entire countries have been changed geographically, economically, and religiously as a result of sweeping virus infections that were impervious to known cures.

Smallpox alone, in the twentieth century, has killed an estimated 300 million individuals, about threefold as many persons as all the wars of this century (1).[*] In the sixteenth and seventeenth centuries, smallpox killed emperors of Japan and Burma, as well as kings and queens of Europe, thereby altering dynasties, control of countries, and alliances (2). Earlier, the successful conquest of Mexican Aztec and Peruvian Inca empires by a handful of Span-

[*]Numbers in parentheses refer to Works Cited at the end of the book.

ish conquistadors led by Hernando Cortés and Francisco Pizarro, respectively, resulted in large part from epidemics of smallpox and measles virus infection that decimated the native defenders. Most of the conquistadors had been exposed to these viruses in Europe, so were immune to (protected from) their effects, but those of the New World were completely vulnerable. In fact, neither the obvious technical superiority of the Spaniards and the superstitions that Quetzalcoatl or other gods would destroy the natives, nor the Spaniards' alliances with tribes subjugated by the Aztecs or Incas accounts for the Spanish victory. History asserts that the Aztecs, once incited to fight, savagely attacked and defeated the Spanish. However, on the very evening that the Aztecs drove the conquistadors out of what is now Mexico City, killing many while routing the rest, a smallpox epidemic began. As it raged in the city (3), not only did the susceptible Aztec forces die in droves, but the psychological aspect of seeing Spaniards, who fought under a Christian god, resist this new malady while warriors of the Aztec gods were dying of infection demoralized the natives even further. The Aztecs could not have known that smallpox was endemic in Europe at this time and that many in Spain exposed to smallpox earlier were resistant or immune to subsequent infection by this virus. The stricken Aztecs interpreted the death of their people while the Spaniards went untouched as a clear indication that the Christian god held dominance over native gods. Therefore, one direct consequence of mass smallpox infection was the subjugation and subsequent exploitation of native Americans and Mexicans by the Spaniards. A second and more lasting effect was destruction of the native culture; as the Spaniard culture assumed sovereignty, millions of Indians were converted to the Christian faith. During the time of the Spanish conquest in the New World it is estimated that more than one-third of the total native population had been killed by smallpox viruses.

In addition to propelling the establishment of Christianity in Mexico and Latin America, viruses played a role in enlarging the African slave trade throughout the Americas. African blacks are relatively resistant to yellow fever virus, whereas Caucasians and native Americans are much more susceptible. Because so many native Americans had died from yellow fever, too few workers remained to do chores in the fields and mines. The Spaniards then imported black slaves as labor replacements (3). The net result was expansion of black slave importation to the Americas (4); ironically, the yellow fever virus initially came from Africa aboard trading and slave ships.

In addition to Spain, other European countries staked out colonies in the Americas. The French colonized Haiti and, in keeping with their observation that the Africans resisted infection by yellow fever and therefore were stronger workers, used primarily black labor for their plantations. But viruses altered human history again when black slaves revolted in the early years of the nineteenth century. To put down that uprising, Napoleon sent over 27,000 crack troops to Haiti. Before long, the vast majority of these French men came in contact with the yellow fever virus transmitted by mosquitos and died from the infection. This huge loss influenced the decision not to risk the even larger numbers of troops necessary to protect other French territories in the New World and was one of the major considerations leading Napoleon to negotiate the sale of the Louisiana Territory to the United States (5).

England also colonized large parts of North America, including what was to become the early United States and Canada. During the Revolutionary War, the American colonial government sent an army to wrest Canada away from the English. Having captured Montreal, the colonial army, superior in numbers, marched on to engage in the conquest of Quebec City. But smallpox entered their ranks. The decimated American army (6), soon after burying their dead in mass graves, retreated in disorder from Quebec.

The bigger picture lies in the after-effects of smallpox, measles, and yellow fever viruses. Some historians link the Spaniards' New World riches with the initial dominance of Spain in Europe. Nevertheless, the later demise of Spain in European politics is attributed by some primarily to wealth acquired from the Americas, which fostered a leisure population that was slow to enter the industrial revolution. The situation may have been very different had the natives not been susceptible to the diseases the Spanish brought over. Viruses interfered so that Canada and the United States never united into a single country. Further, the virus-promoted Louisiana Purchase provided an opportunity for the United States to enhance its size by unprecedented western expansion, without precipitating a potential geo-political conflict with France. The aftermath of virus infection uprooted native cultures and peoples of south, central, and Latin America and replaced them with a European culture, where Christianity flourished. Enhanced transport and introduction of black African slaves in the New World filled a niche created by yellow fever viruses.

But at that time, who would have imagined that the ancient diseases of humankind, smallpox and measles, would eventually be controlled? Smallpox, after decimating the ancient Mexican population, still continued to kill, for example, until the early 1940s, being responsible for the deaths of over 10,000 Mexicans a year. Yet smallpox has now been eradicated not only from Mexico but also from the entire world as a result of vaccination programs. Eradication of measles virus is also a reasonable goal in view of its control in most industrialized countries. In 1970, measles viruses infected an estimated 130 million individuals and nearly killed eight million. Today in the underdeveloped countries of the Third World, measles virus infects about 40 million individuals per year with a death rate approaching one million.

Poliomyelitis virus is a relatively new virus. Polio epidemics were not recorded until the nineteenth century, followed by an increasing incidence in the twentieth century (7). At one time, poliomyelitis virus infection was responsible for one-fifth of the deaths from acute disease in Sweden (8). No one would have guessed then that poliomyelitis would now be under control or that its eradication from this planet would be a goal of the World Health Organization for the year 2000. Similarly, because of vaccination, yellow fever virus no longer spreads the havoc and fear it once did. These triumphs of medicine reflect the achievements that are possible when medical scientists and government agencies together devote their resources to solving health problems.

In contrast with these harnessed viruses, new plagues of fearful proportions have now appeared. Human immunodeficiency virus (HIV) is currently reported to infect nearly 100 million people. There is no satisfactory treatment to permanently arrest the disease. There is no vaccine to prevent it. There are no known spontaneous cures.

Other plagues are now also emerging. Hemorrhagic fevers made their formidable appearance in the second half of the twentieth century. Evident on all continents, exhibiting frightening death rates, they claim numerous victims. Ebola, Hanta, and Lassa viruses provoke the fear today that yellow fever, poliomyelitis, and smallpox did in previous times. One former plague, a type of influenza virus that killed over 20 million persons between 1918 and 1919—more victims than died in World War I—may make a comeback.

Last in this list is the current scare that beef from cattle with mad cow disease is causing human dementia. However, both the probability of an epidemic and identification of the causative agent as a virus remain debatable.

To assist the reader in understanding how plagues of the past were first observed and then controlled, despite numerous difficulties, the next two chapters briefly review the principles of virus infection and its course. Chapter 2 defines what a virus is, how it replicates, and how it causes disease. The third chapter explores how the human immune system combats viruses, either aborting infections or becoming stimulated via vaccination to prevent viral diseases. For those interested in virology and immunology, Chapters 2 and 3 are recommended. Otherwise, the reader may skip directly to Chapter 4. Knowing how vaccines were envisioned and developed helps to explain why devising a vaccine for HIV is so difficult, and what steps are required in successfully attacking and combatting a virus infection. The balance of power between any virus and the host it infects reflects the strength, or virulence, of the virus and the resistance or susceptibility of the host.

Readers of this book will encounter the major personalities who became microbe hunters in the fight against smallpox, measles, yellow fever, poliomyelitis, Lassa fever, Ebola, Hantaviruses, HIV, influenza, and spongiform encephalopathies. The history of viruses and virology is also the history of men and women who have worked to combat these diseases. The conquest or control of any disease requires the efforts of many. However, several who became prominent by identifying, isolating, or curing viral infections have been singled out by history as heroes. This book also examines the research of medical investigators which eventually linked certain diseases with specific viruses and led to their ultimate control. Because these scientists—virologists—are human, inevitable conflicts arose among them, and some of these stories are also told.

The history of virology would be incomplete without describing the politics and the superstitions evoked by viruses and the diseases they cause. For example, armed private citizens and militias attempted to prevent frightened crowds from fleeing Memphis in 1878–79 during an epidemic of yellow fever, from leaving New York City in 1916 because of poliomyelitis, and from abandoning Zwitheba, Zaire (renamed Congo Republic in 1997), in 1995 to escape Ebola. Thus woven into the fabric of the history of viral plagues is the fear, superstition, and ignorance of man. Further, we can consider together how the people of a country like the United States could unite in a crusade to prevent poliomyelitis, yet succumb to controversy in alleviating the spread of and suffering from HIV. Believe it or not, a similar lack of support by industrialized countries of the world, including the United States, once halted the initial plans to eradicate smallpox (1).

CHAPTER 2

INTRODUCTION TO THE PRINCIPLES OF VIROLOGY

Peter Medawar, a biologist awarded the Nobel Prize for Medicine and Physiology in 1960, defined viruses as a piece of nucleic acid surrounded by bad news (1). True, viruses are nothing more than a speck of genetic material—a single kind of nucleic acid (segmented or nonsegmented, DNA or RNA) and a coat made of protein molecules. Viruses multiply according to the information contained in this nucleic acid. Everything other than the DNA or RNA is dispensable and serves primarily to ensure that the viral nucleic acid gets to the right part of the right sort of cell in the organism hosting the virus, because viruses cannot multiply until they invade a living cell. Viruses enter all cellular forms of life from plants and animals to bacteria, fungi, and protozoa. Viruses, plants, and animals form the three main groups that encompass all living things. Plants and animals are cellular organisms and include bacteria and protozoa. Viruses lack cell walls, are obligatory parasites, and depend for replication on the cells they infect.

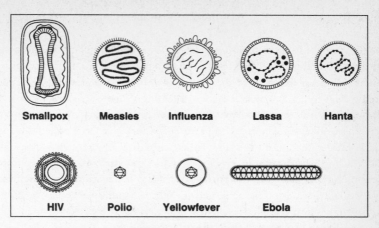

Smallpox   Measles   Influenza   Lassa   Hanta

HIV   Polio   Yellowfever   Ebola

Figure 2.1 Viruses have differing life styles and have evolved a variety of shapes and sizes in which to place their genetic material. A scaled comparison of the various viruses discussed in this book is shown. Viruses vary from the smallest, poliovirus, to the largest, smallpox virus.

Viruses have relatively few genes compared with other organisms. Measles virus, yellow fever virus, poliomyelitis virus, Lassa fever virus, Ebola virus, Hantavirus, as well as the human immunodeficiency virus (HIV), have fewer than ten genes each, whereas a smallpox virus may contain between 200 and 400 genes. These numbers compare with 5,000 to 10,000 genes for the smallest bacteria and approximately 80,000 to 100,000 genes for a human.

It has been argued that the nucleic acid of viruses evolved from normal cell genes. Through the alterations of mutation, reassortment, and recombination, viruses could then have evolved their own genetic structure. Perhaps some viruses stayed within the parental host from which they evolved and displayed symbiotic or near-symbiotic relationships. But as viruses moved from one host species to another or mutated to form new genetic mixtures, these formerly symbiotic viruses may have achieved a high level of virulence. Researchers suspect that the canine distemper virus of dogs or rindepest virus of sheep may have crossed species to enter humans in whom they mutated sufficiently to become measles virus. This is postulated because the genomic sequences of canine distemper virus, rindepest virus, and measles virus have more in common than do sequences from other types of viruses. Such interrelationships between these three viruses likely occurred at the time when large human populations first lived in close proximity to domestic animals. A similar event may have enabled simian (monkey) viruses to infect humans, become HIV, and cause AIDS. In fact, whenever a virus encounters an unfamiliar organism, the virus may undergo multiple mutations and emerge as a variant that produces a severe and novel disease.

To maintain itself in nature and to replicate, a virus must undergo a series of steps. First, the virus contacts the cell to be infected and then attaches to its surface. A major function of the plasma membrane or outer "skin" of nucleated cells is to act as a barrier against infecting viruses. Yet viruses often cross through this membrane to carry their genetic material and accessory proteins into the cell's cytosol (inner compartment). Next, the virus penetrates to the cell's interior, leading to the uncoating or removal of the virus's outer husk. Thereafter, the virus uses its evolved strategies to express its genes, replicate its genome (genes placed in the correct order and orientation), and assemble its component parts (nucleic acids and proteins) in multiple copies or progeny (offspring). Upon completion of this sequence, mature viruses formed during the replication process exit from the infected cell.

Generally, the attachment and entry of viruses into cells are dependent both on the activities of the host cell and on the properties of selected viral genes. The cell has on its surface receptors to which viruses attach and bind with proteins evolved specifically for that purpose. The cell must also provide the mechanism for viral penetration after binding has occurred, and for the internal highway that viruses travel to reach sites in the cell's cytoplasm or nucleus where replication processes can proceed.

As described above, the attachment or binding of a viral protein (specifically, an amino acid sequence within that protein) to a cell receptor is the first step that initiates infection of a cell. The unique distribution of certain receptors and either their limitation to a few cell types or, instead, their broad range on many different cell types dictate how many portals of entry exist for a virus. Further, the type of cells with such receptors and/or with the ability to replicate a given virus often determines the severity of illness that a virus can cause and the distribution of areas (organs, tissues, cells) in the body affected, and the host's potential for recovery. For example, infections of neuronal cells in the central nervous system that are not replaceable or of cells of the heart whose function is essential to life are more ominous than infection of skin cells which are less critical to survival and are replaceable.

An example of a cellular receptor is a molecule called CD4, which is abundant on the surfaces of some lymphocytes (white blood cells) derived from the thymus ($CD4^+$ T cells). The CD4 molecule is also present, but less plentiful, on monocyte macrophages (macrophages are infection fighting cells, an activated form of monocytes) in the blood and in certain tissues of the body. The CD4 molecule along with certain chemokine (cell-attracting) molecules is the receptor for HIV. Because the CD4 receptor appears on relatively few cell types that HIV can infect, these viruses attack only limited sites in the body (2,3). By contrast, a molecule called CD46, the cell receptor for measles virus, appears on many types of cells (4–7). CD46 is found on epithelial cells, which line most cavities including the nose, pharynx, respiratory tree, and gut; on endothelial cells lining blood vessels; on lymphocytes/macrophages; and on neuronal cells in the brain. The common presence of the CD46 receptors correlates with the widespread replication of measles virus during infection.

In addition to access through specific cell receptors, viruses can enter cells by other means. When a foreign agent composed of foreign proteins (antigens) such as a virus enters the body, a defensive response by the host produces antibodies that bind to the antigen in an attempt to remove it. Because antibodies are shaped roughly like the letter "Y," they can bind to cells in two ways. First, via their arms (the two upper parts of the "Y"), antibodies use a combining site (the so-called FAb'2 site) to interact specifically with antigens on cells. Second, with a part of their stalk (the bottom part of the "Y") called the F_c region, antibody molecules can bind to receptors (F_c receptors) on certain cells. After antibodies made by the host's immune system against viral antigens bind to those antigens an infectious virus–antibody complex forms (8). By binding to the cell via the F_c receptor, the virus as part of the virus–antibody complex can enter that cell even though its surface may not contain a specific receptor for the virus.

Not all cells that bind and take in a virus have the appropriate machinery to replicate that virus. Therefore, binding to a receptor and entry of a virus into a cell may not result in production of progeny. To summarize, the susceptibility of a specific cell for a virus is dependent on at least three factors. First, a functional receptor must be present on the cell. Second, a specific viral protein, or sequence within the protein, must be available to bind to the cell receptor. Third, the cell must possess the correct machinery to assist in replication of the virus.

The post-binding step in which viruses can penetrate a cell is an active process and depends on energy. Occurring within seconds of binding/attachment, penetration follows either by movement of the entire virus across the cell's plasma membrane, a process called phagocytosis (more specifically, endocytosis), so that the virus particle is pinched off inside a vacuole or compartment of the cell, or by fusion of the cell's membrane with the virus's outer envelope. After penetration, the virus sheds its protective protein coat and then releases its viral nucleic acids. This procedure is followed by replication of the viral genome, during which the host cell's protein manufacturing equipment actually synthesizes new viruses—their progeny. To produce abundant amounts of their own proteins, viruses must evolve strategies that provide advantages for synthesizing viral materials instead of host cells' materials. Viruses accomplish this feat either by abolishing the cell's ability to make its own products or by conferring a selective advantage for the making of viral products.

Whatever the route, once the viral genome and proteins form, they assemble as multiple progeny viruses, they mature, and they leave the infected cell. Individual viruses have evolved unique processes and "patented" them for success in this process. Once formed as a mature particle, viruses display distinctive sizes and shapes.

How do viruses cause disease? Three distinct pathways are available (9, 10). By the first, the virus or its proteins are directly toxic to a cell. In this instance, the virus kills its host cell. With some viruses this process serves to release virus particles from the inside of a cell to the outside environment. Alternatively, a second mechanism enables a virus to avoid killing the cell but instead to alter its function. By this means, the synthesis of an important product made by a cell is turned down or turned up. For example, a nonlethal virus infection of cells that make growth hormone can diminish the amount of this hormone made by the infected host cell. As a result the host fails to grow and develop normally. The third way in which injury and disease can follow a viral infection is through the participation of the host's immune response. As stated in Chapter 3, the immune response to viruses is generated to rid infected cells of virus progeny and to remove infectious virus from the host's blood and other body fluids. By destroying virally infected cells, the immune system can damage tissues that are critical to healthy function of the organism. Additionally, virus–antibody immune complexes can form that subsequently can be deposited or become trapped in kidneys and blood vessels, which are then injured. Thus, another side of the usually protective immune response is its destructive potential. The study of such processes is called immunopathology. The balance between the protective and destructive processes of the immune system is in large part responsible for the clinical symptoms (what the patient states he or she has) and signs (what the doctor finds) that accompany a virus infection.

How were viruses recognized as dangers to health? Although the diseases caused by viruses were known in antiquity, viruses were not acknowledged as separate infectious agents until about a hundred years ago, in the late 1890s.

The mid-1800s were the time of the discovery of bacteria and the pioneering work of Louis Pasteur, Robert Koch, and their associates. During that period, the laboratory culturing process was developed so that bacteria could be grown at will, then fixed on glass slides, stained, and observed under the microscope. Bacteria were retained on filters with specific pore sizes, which

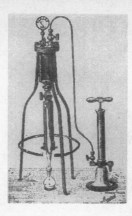

Figure 2.2 The Pasteur-Chamberland type filter connected to a hand pump and used at the Pasteur Institute toward the end of the nineteenth century.

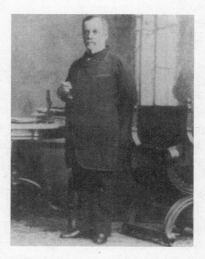

Figure 2.3 Louis Pasteur, who, with Robert Koch, founded the discipline of microbiology. Pasteur also attenuated (reduced virulence in) several infectious agents, including rabies virus, to make vaccines.

allowed calculation of a bacterium's size. After their identification, specific bacteria could be linked with particular disease states. This was the framework in which the first viruses were uncovered. Just before the current century began, Dmitri Iosifovich Ivanovski (11) in Russia and Martinus Beijerinck (12) in the Netherlands demonstrated that the material responsible for a dis-

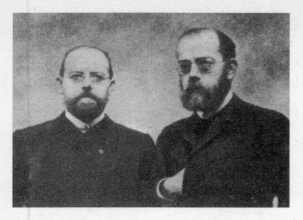

Figure 2.4 Friedrich Loeffler (right) and his teacher and mentor Robert Koch (left), who with Louis Pasteur created the field of microbiology. Loeffler and Paul Frosch isolated the first animal virus, foot-and-mouth virus, in 1898. The virus was separated from bacteria by its ability to pass through a Pasteur-Chamberland filter.

ease of tobacco plants instead of being retained passed through the pores of a Pasteur–Chamberland filter without losing infectivity. The investigators found that this soluble residue of filtration could somehow grow on healthy tobacco leaves. Their result was the first report of a plant virus, the tobacco mosaic virus. Similarly, Friedrich Loeffler and Paul Frosch (13) in Germany concluded that the agent causing foot-and-mouth disease of cows also passed through porcelain filters and induced symptoms of disease when inoculated into previously healthy cattle. These observations, highly controversial at the time, provided the basis for defining viruses as subcellular entities that could cause distinct forms of tissue destruction, which became marks of specific diseases.

Most viral infections are recognized as an acute illness. That is, the causative virus enters the body, multiplies in one or more tissues, and spreads locally through the blood or along nerves. The incubation period of two days to two or three weeks is followed by signs and symptoms of disease and local or widespread tissue damage. Viruses can be isolated from the patient's blood (serum or blood cells) or secretions for a short time just before and after the appearance of symptoms. Afterward, the infected host either recovers from the infection and is often blessed with life-long immunity to that virus, or dies during the acute phase of illness.

Distinct from acute infections are persistent infections in which the immune response fails to completely remove viruses from the body, and those

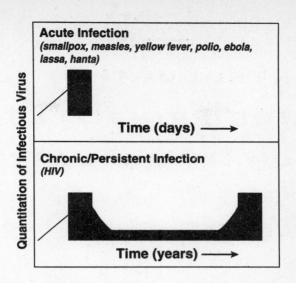

Figure 2.5 Infections caused by viruses differ. Some are acute and the outcome is decided within a week or two. Others, like HIV, routinely run a years-long infectious course in the human host. The darkened area indicates the presence of virus.

remaining persist for months or years. As in the case of HIV infection, viruses can be recovered for years throughout the long course of infection. Although all components (antibodies and T cells) of the immune response are generated during HIV infection, and for a considerable period of time the amount of virus load is markedly reduced, the response is not capable of terminating the infection. Then, during the terminal stage of the illness, T-cell immunity declines or vanishes and a high viral load recurs. Figure 2.5 shows the differences between acute and persistent infection. How the immune response is constituted and how it attacks viruses are described in the next chapter.

CHAPTER 3

INTRODUCTION TO THE PRINCIPLES OF IMMUNOLOGY

A misunderstanding of the term "immunity" has arisen because the general public usually interprets immunity to mean the ability to avoid a disease, but the medical scientist knows that infection does occur, although in a mild form that precludes serious or life-threatening consequences. Antigens are the proteins in viruses and bacteria that trigger an immune response, and the result of a satisfactory immune response is immunity—protection from repeated disease caused by a specific type of virus or bacteria (1).

The immune system has evolved to deal with enormous numbers and varieties of every conceivable foreign substance, that is, antigen. A consequence of virus entry and replication in an organism—the host—is the manufacture of viral antigens that, in most cases, elicit an immune response by that host. Success of this system defines an organism's capacity for survival. In addition, the immune system must discriminate between foreign antigens, such as viral proteins, that are nonself and those antigens that are self, one's own proteins (i.e., hormones such as insulin and cell proteins that make up muscle).

After an initial exposure to viral infection, or the acute phase, a race is on between the virus, which is replicating rapidly, and the host's immune system, which functions first to limit the amount of virus made and second to clear the virus from the host. At stake is whether the virus can successfully replicate itself. To combat the virus, the host mobilizes and uses many weapons, both immunologically specific and nonspecific responses. The nonspecific factors are all early combatants against the virus and the cells it infects. Included in this group are natural killer lymphoid cells, phagocytic macrophages—large cells that ingest or eat viruses—and proteins in the blood called complement factors that are capable of interacting with viruses and also destroying cells. However, the major combatants against viruses are those involved in the specific immune response, particularly antibodies and T lymphocytes (defined below). These components are preconditioned by vaccines to have a ready and rapid start when the host is first exposed to virus infection (1). For small-pox, measles, yellow fever, poliomyelitis, the hemorrhagic fever and influenza viruses, the generation of antigen-specific immune responses by antibodies, CD4T cells, and cytotoxic T lymphocytes (CTLs) terminates the infection. The specific host immune response against viruses is mounted by both antibodies and CTLs.

A clearly defined winner in the race between a virus and its host is often decided in less than ten to fourteen days. If the immune response wins, the viruses are vanquished, and the host survives with enduring immunity to that virus.

However, if the immune response is overcome, the acute viral infection ends in either death of the host or a chronic-persistent infection. During chronic-persistent infection, the time scale of disease is lengthened, and ongoing viral replication can continue despite an immune response that, by definition in this situation, is ineffective in terminating the infection and clearing the virus. In contrast to the short duration of acute infection, this longer-term scenario plays out during HIV infection, for example.

The course of HIV infection is as follows. Soon after HIV enters a host's cells and replicates there, a vigorous immune response generates CTLs, and this response correlates directly with a decrease in the host's viral load. An antibody response is also generated, although it appears for the most part after reduction of the viral load. Reduced but not eliminated are the key words, because even the combined vigorous CTL and antibody responses fail to terminate HIV infection. Instead, anti-HIV CTLs as well as anti-HIV antibodies now coexist with the virus. Later in the course of HIV infection, the anti-HIV CTLs lose effectiveness, the viral load increases, and the patient approaches death. The loss of CTL activity late in HIV infection likely results from the increasing loss of CD4 helper/inducer cells, cells that are believed necessary to help maintain CTL activity over prolonged periods of time, and, perhaps in part by newly generated virus variants that escape CTL recognition. In contrast, in acute infection a vigorous CTL and antibody response removes all the virus.

Vaccination is the medical strategy for stimulating the immune system to protect against a specific disease agent prior to exposure. Provoking an immune response before a natural viral infection occurs acts to "blueprint" immunologic memory so that cells involved in making the potential antiviral immune response are primed and held alert. When confronted with the full-strength infectious virus, these primed cells react quickly and with greater intensity than unprimed cells, thus enhancing the host's ability to successfully combat and control the infection.

Historically, three different routes have been taken in developing antiviral vaccines. The first employs "live virus" vaccines. These are usually prepared by passage in a laboratory animal and tissue culture or in tissue culture alone, which decreases the disease-causing ability of virus. This process, called attenuation, yields a form of the virus with just enough potency to cause an immune response but not enough to cause disease. This attenuated, live virus is then tested initially in animal models and later in human volunteers. This was the method followed for the successful smallpox, measles, yellow fever, and Sabin poliomyelitis vaccines. By the second route, the virulent virus is inactivated, essentially killed, by use of a chemical such as formalin. The killed virus is then tested for its capacity to cause an immune response as above. The Salk poliomyelitis virus vaccine is a successful example of this approach. The third option is preparation of a subunit, recombinant, or DNA vaccine. The successful hepatitis B virus vaccine is an example of a recombinant vaccine; other subunit and DNA vaccines are currently under experimental analysis but have not had sufficient testing in clinical trials for general use.

Cells process live viruses differently than killed viruses. Processing of their antigens by cells follows two distinct pathways called class I and class II (1). For the class I pathway, antigens inside cells from living, replicating viruses (virulent or attenuated) are broken into smaller components called peptides. According to several physical–chemical parameters, some of these antigenic peptides bind to grooves within host proteins (called major histocompatibility complex (MHC) class I proteins), then travel to and wait on cells' surfaces to be recognized by CTLs that react with a CD8 receptor (CD8$^+$). The class II pathway primarily handles antigens that are initially outside the cell. These antigens (usually killed viruses, or toxins) enter the cell (endocytosis) via phagocytosis, and the protein is broken down into peptides inside vesicles where it then binds to the host's proteins (called MHC class II proteins). The complex is then presented on the surface of a cell to await recognition by CD4$^+$ T cells (as described in Chapter 2). To summarize, the key is the location where the antigen ends up. Viral antigens synthesized inside cells join to MHC class I proteins, whereas those captured outside cells attach to MHC class II proteins. Although this division is not absolute, it is an accurate generalization. In general, vaccines made from killed viruses do not necessarily induce a good CD8$^+$ CTL response, and the immunity so induced is not as long-lasting as in the case of attenuated live vaccine.

What are these CD8$^+$ and CD4$^+$ T cells? The T stands for thymus-derived and CD8$^+$ or CD4$^+$ indicate specific molecules on their surfaces. The thymus is a two-lobed gland of the lymphoid system located over the heart and under the breastbone. Lymphocytes formed in the bone marrow (hemopoietic stem cells) travel to and enter the thymus where they are educated (mature) and are then selected to become either CD8$^+$ or CD4$^+$ T cells. CD8$^+$ T cells function as surveillance and killer cells, which accounts for their name "cytotoxic T lymphocytes" (CTLs). They travel along the highways of blood vessels and wander among tissues throughout the body seeking cells that are foreign (not like self) because they express viral proteins or are transformed by cancers. CD8$^+$ CTLs then recognize, attack, and kill such cells. CD4$^+$ T cells usually serve a different role. They release soluble materials (proteins) that help or induce bone marrow-derived (non-thymic-educated) B lymphocytes to differentiate and make antibodies. CD4$^+$ T lymphocytes also assist CD8$^+$ T lymphocytes and macrophages, prompting their designation as helper/inducer T cells (1–5). They also release soluble factors (cytokines) that also participate in clearing a virus infection.

T lymphocytes use their cell surface receptors to interact with protein fragments or peptides of the viral antigen. T cells interact with viral peptides attached to MHC molecules on the surfaces of infected cells. These MHC proteins actually carry the viral peptides to cells' surfaces. Thus T lymphocytes seek foreign antigens (in this case, viral antigens—peptides derived from the viral protein) on the surfaces of infected cells being parasitized by the virus. Once the T cell recognizes that the infected cell is "foreign" (contains virus), it becomes activated and either directly kills the infected cell and/or releases soluble factors (lymphokines, cytokines) that alert and arm other cells of the host to join the battle. In addition, some of these cytokines can directly interfere with viral replication (1,3–5). By such means, the spread of viruses is inhibited, and the nidus of infection removed.

Antibody and CTL responses rely on lymphocytes, which originate from hemopoietic stem cells during the blood-forming process (2). Antibodies and

CTLs represent the two arms of antigen-specific immune responses, and both play important roles in combatting infection. There is a built-in plasticity to overall immunity such that the relative contribution of each arm of the immune response varies according to the infecting virus. Antibodies primarily react with viruses in the body fluids and are, therefore, most effective in limiting the spread of virus through the blood or in cerebrospinal fluids that bathe the brain and spinal cord. By this means antibodies decrease a host's content of virus and diminish infectivity, thereby lowering the numbers of infected cells. However, the eradication of virus-infected cells and their removal is the primary job of the CTLs. By removing infected cells, CTLs eliminate the factories that manufacture viral progeny. As the number of virus particles released is reduced, the work of antibodies becomes easier.

Antibodies are large protein molecules. They latch onto and neutralize viruses by one of several mechanisms: (1) Antibodies can coat or block the outer spike protein of the virus that attaches to receptors on a cell and initiates viral entry into the cell; (2) antibodies can aggregate or clump viruses so that the net number of infectious particles is reduced; and (3) with the assistance of complement, a group of proteins in the blood, antibodies can lyse (disintegrate) viruses (6). Each antibody molecule generated acts on a specific antigen or target molecule of the virus. The host has the capacity to synthesize billions of different antibodies via genes that dictate their manufacture.

Antibodies are made by B lymphocytes, named for their source, the bone marrow (2). B lymphocytes are small resting lymphocytes with nuclei that virtually fill these cells; little cytoplasm is present. When a virus or viral protein is encountered by a specific lymphocyte with a preconceived receptor for the antibody that matches the virus's protein structure, the lymphocyte becomes stimulated to divide and the amount of cytoplasm composing the cell's volume increases. The expanded cytoplasm factory then manufactures antibodies designed to interact with the virus that stimulated their production and exports these antibody molecules into the immediate milieu. One such activated B lymphocyte can pump out 100 million antiviral antibody molecules per hour.

CD4$^+$ T cells can in some specialized instances also function as cytotoxic cells. Conversely, the CD8$^+$ cells can release soluble molecules so they also have a helper/inducer activity, although their primary function is to recognize and destroy virus-infected cells. One CD8$^+$ CTL can kill five or more virally infected cells in as short a time as two minutes. Further, these CTLs can recognize viral peptides on infected cells before virus particles are assembled and thus effectively and efficiently kill these cells before viral progeny are produced.

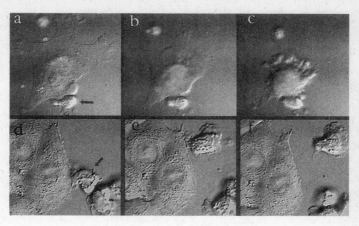

Figure 3.1 Lysis of a virus-infected cell by cytotoxic T lymphocytes (CTLs)(a–c) The steps of a virus-infected cell being killed. (a) The arrow points to a CTL bound to the infected cell. In c, the virus-infected cell has shrunk and developed blisters or ballooned areas. This cell is dead. This sequence of events occurs in less than two minutes. Bar, 14 μm. (d–f) The binding of a CTL to a target cell that CTLs cannot kill. The time sequence of d to f is over thirty minutes. Bar, 8 μm. Photomicrographs by Klaus Hahn and Michael B. A. Oldstone.

When the host is initially exposed to an infecting virus or to a vaccine containing viral antigens, both viral antibodies and CTLs are generated. The CTL response is strong within five days after the exposure, peaks on the seventh to tenth day, and decreases after the resolution of infection. Antibody responses peak after the CTL response, and unattached or free antibodies are often weakly detectable during the acute phase of infection. The number of antibodies then rises over a period of two to four weeks following infection, and they linger for years. B cells as well as T cells can be memory cells, that is, cells that previously have seen a particular virus. Such memory cells frequently last for the host's entire lifetime and function to protect the host from reinfection with the same virus (4). This is the scenario played out in those who survive infection from smallpox, measles, yellow fever, poliomyelitis, or hemorrhagic fever viruses.

With a persistent virus infection like HIV, the immune response fails to clear the viruses, since they, too, have evolved protective mechanisms. The genes that all viruses carry have one of two primary functions. One group of genes ensures the replication of viral progeny. These genes encode proteins that protect the virus from harsh conditions during its transport from one

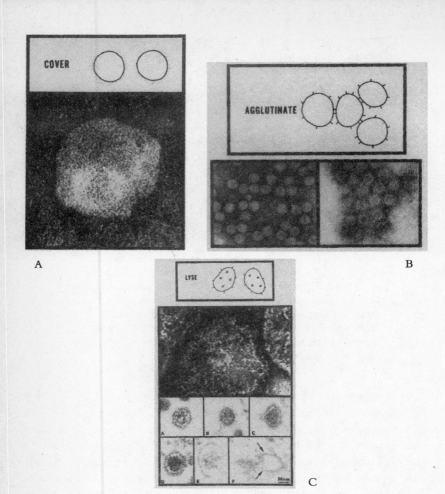

Figure 3.2 Antibodies can, with or without the complement proteins in the blood, blanket virus particles (A, action of antibody on coronavirus), clump together viral particles (B, action of antibody on polyomavirus); and with the participation of complement, directly destroy the virus (C, top, retrovirus; C, bottom, arenavirus). Lysis of the retrovirus produces holes (arrows), but lysis of the arenavirus begins a progression of events climaxing in the release of virus nucleic acids to the outside environment away from the protective virus coat. Photomicrographs modified from Michael B.A. Oldstone, "Virus Neutralization and Virus-Induced Immune Complex Disease: Virus-Antibody Union Resulting in Immunoprotection or Immunologic Injury—Two Sides of the Same Coin," Progr. Med.Virol. *19(1975):84–119.*

host to the next; that is, they stabilize the infectious particle for travel through the environment. Also encoded are viral proteins that bind the virus to its receptors on cells, assist in internalization of the virus into cells, and provide the appropriate signaling for replication, assembly, and exit of the virus progeny from the parasitized cell. The second group of genes has among its main purposes the subjugation and/or modification of a host's immune system. By such strategies the virus can manipulate the normal function of the immune system to escape surveillance and destruction for itself and the cells it infects. The outcome is the persistence of viruses within their living host.

PART TWO

SUCCESS
STORIES

CHAPTER 4

SMALLPOX

Smallpox, which killed nearly 300 million people in the twentieth century alone—three times more than all the wars in this century—has been eradicated (1,2). The story of this most universally feared disease and of its elimination is the topic of this chapter. Yet one of the more interesting notes about this major accomplishment of mankind is that considerable opposition stood in the way of its conquest two hundred years ago, as well as in the recent past.

The story of smallpox is interwoven with the history of human migrations and wars, dramatically favoring one population or army over another. Smallpox actually changed the course of history by killing generals and kings or decimating their enemies.

The smallpox virus has no animal reservoir; its infection is limited to humans (3). Subclinical, or medically undetectable, infections are rare, if they occur at all. The typical course of smallpox is an acute disease that produces obvious and distinct skin lesions and after recovery leaves its well-defined fingerprints as clearly visible, distinctive pock marks, usually numerous, on the

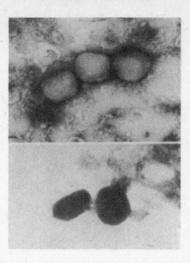

Figure 4.1 Smallpox virus obtained from fluid of a human smallpox vesicle. Bar, 100 nm. Photomicrograph from E. L. Palmer and M. L. Martin, An Atlas of Mammalian Viruses *(1982), courtesy of CRC Press, Inc.*

faces of survivors. After an incubation period of ten to fourteen days during which the infected subject is well and mobile, fever, weakness, and headache suddenly begin, followed in two to three days by the distinctive rash. With the appearance of the rash, the patient becomes infectious, as lesions on the mucosal membranes allow viruses to be spread through the air. Skin-to-skin contact is less important as a route of spreading the infection. Therefore, people in small, isolated communities can avoid contact with the smallpox virus, but once it is introduced, the effects are devastating.

How smallpox evolved as an infectious agent and when it first infected man are unclear (1,3–7). The virus probably made its appearance as the first agricultural settlements were being established in 10,000 B.C. along the great river basins. The earliest hint of smallpox infection is the extensive lesions found on three Egyptian mummies, the most renowned being Ramses V. We know that Ramses died of an acute illness in 1157 B.C., his fortieth year of life. When his mummified remains were discovered in 1898, his face and neck displayed a striking rash of pustules strongly resembling smallpox. Other ancient plagues considered to result from smallpox (1,3–7) were recorded in 1346 B.C. by the Hittites, in 595 B.C. in Syracuse, in 490 B.C. in Athens, in 48 A.D. in China, in 583 A.D. in the Korean Peninsula, and in 585 A.D. in Japan. Ho Kung, a Chinese medical writer (A.D. 281–361) wrote

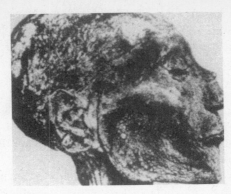

Figure 4.2 Mummy of Ramses V, who died in his early thirties probably from smallpox in 1158 B.C. Smallpox lesions are visible on his lower face and neck.

Recently there have been persons suffering from epidemic sores which attack the head, face, and trunk. In a short time, these sores spread all over the body. They have the appearance of hard boils containing white matter. While some of the pustules are drying up, a fresh crop appears. If not treated early the patients usually die. Those who recover are disfigured by purplish scars (on the face) which do not fade until after a year.

The lack of any written description of the rash and the inability of physicians of antiquity to distinguish the rash of smallpox from other skin rashes like measles, however, makes these diagnoses suggestive rather than definitive.

In A.D. 570, an army from Abyssinia (now Ethiopia) attacked the Arabic capital of Mecca for the purpose of destroying the Kaaba and subjugating the native population. The Kaaba was a shrine sacred to the Arabs, who at this time were not yet Moslems. According to the Koran, God sent flocks of birds that showered the attacking armies with stones, producing sores and pustules that spread like a pestilence. The Abyssinian troops soon became decimated and Abraha, their leader, died from the disease. This war was recorded in the Koran:

> *In the name of Allah, the Beneficent, the Merciful,*
> *Hast thou not seen how the Lord dealt with the possessors of the elephant*
> *[Ahraha arrived mounted on a white elephant]*
> *Did He not cause their wars to end in confusion?*
> *And send against them birds in flocks?*
> *Casting at them decreed stones—*
> *So He rendered them like straw eaten up?*

Coincidentally, the year A.D. 570 was also the birth year of Mohammed, the prophet of Islam. By 622, Ad Ahrun, a Christian priest living in Alexandria, described the pox lesion, and in 910 the Arab physician Al-Razi descriptively separated the skin rash of smallpox from that caused by measles in his patients (9).

The great Islamic expansion across North Africa and into the Iberian Peninsula in the sixth through eighth centuries spread smallpox across Africa and into Europe. This migration was defined by the Saracens' (now known as Moors) capture of Tripoli in 647, the invasion of Spain in 710, and crossing of the Pyrenees to invade France in 731.

By 1000, smallpox epidemics had been recorded in populated areas from Japan to Spain and throughout African countries on the southern rim of the Mediterranean Sea. The eleventh to thirteenth centuries abounded with the movement of people to and from Asia Minor during the Crusades (1096–1291) and of African caravans crossing the Sahara to West Africa and the port cities of East Africa, carrying smallpox as well as goods.

By the sixteenth century, multiple smallpox outbreaks in European countries were reflected by statistics then being collected in several large cities including London, Geneva, and Stockholm. Because the sixteenth century was a time of exploration, often on ocean-going ships, smallpox was spread across oceans by mariners as well as over land routes by armies and caravans (3). These European explorers, and the colonists who soon followed to the newly discovered continents of America, Australia, and South Africa, brought smallpox as part of their baggage. Indeed, the inadvertent arrival of smallpox played a crucial role in the Spanish conquest of Mexico and Peru, the Portuguese colonization of Brazil, the settlement of North America by the English and French, as well as the settlements of Australia.

In the Americas, the decimation of native Indian populations made both conquest and colonization easier (10). The native population, initially considered by the conquistadors and church as not having souls, therefore being not human but similar to animals, were worked in mines and plantations as beasts of burden. Such inhuman working conditions, coupled with diseases brought from Europe, reduced the labor pool available. With so much of the native Indian labor force lost, the impetus grew to bring slaves from West African ports as replacements. This was especially so in Hispaniola (now the Dominican Republic) and Cuba, stimulating, in large part, the establishment of slave trade to the New World. The epidemic of smallpox began in the New World with an outbreak in Hispaniola, and by 1518 it had killed many of the native population. By 1519, the plague had spread to Cuba. By 1520 smallpox occupied the Yucatan and other parts of Mexico (10).

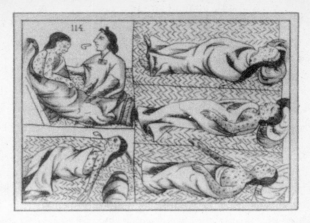

*Figure 4.3 Smallpox victims in this sixteenth-century Aztec drawing
from the Códue Florentino.*

Hernando Cortés, initially with less than 500 conquistadors and followers,
set out to explore and claim the territory of the Yucatan and other parts of
Mexico for the King of Spain. At that time, in the early 1500s, the Aztecs
ruled over Mexico, forcing many tribes into submission and obtaining tribute
from them. With an elaborate system of messengers and roads, their emperor,
Montezuma, was kept up to date on the landings and movements of Cortés
from the isle of Cozumel in the Yucatan to the east and north until he
reached what is now Veracruz. Cortés shrewdly convinced a number of native
tribes to become his allies by promising to remove the yoke of Aztec domina-
tion. He was favored in this endeavor by the legend of Quetzalcoatl, a god
predicted to arrive from the east on the wind and destroy the Aztec empire.
Cortés must have seemed like the living manifestation of this legend, arriving
from the east in boats with sails. Cortés and his men, because their landing
was on Good Friday, were dressed in black, one of Quetzalcoatl's fabled col-
ors. The Spaniards were themselves of a different (lighter) complexion than
the natives, and wore beards, so might even resemble the god. Finally, the
Spaniards rode horses and brought attack dogs as well as cannons and rifles,
materials of war never seen before by natives. With the abundance of such
unfavorable signs, Montezuma decided to appease Cortés and his followers
when they reached Tenochtitlan (now Mexico City), the capital of the Aztec
empire. Yet in reality, the Spanish were greatly outnumbered. Later, when the
Aztecs united under Montezuma's brother Cuitlahuac, his cousin Cuauhte-
moc, and other nobles, they fought the Spaniards and, after inflicting heavy
casualties on the Spaniards, forced their retreat to a coastal settlement. The

Spaniards had lost nearly one-third of their men, and their defeat on the bridges of Tenochtitlan was the biggest loss suffered until then by Europeans. If the Aztecs had continued their pursuit, the Europeans would have been expelled from Mexico. But the Aztecs did not. Why did they not follow up their initial victory and annihilate the remaining Spaniards?

The answer, by a devious route, lies in the appearance of smallpox. Diego Velázquez, the governor of Cuba and rival of Cortés, had initially but hesitantly sent Cortés on his mission to Mexico. Not only had Velázquez been suspicious of Cortés's ambition but he also wanted the power and the riches of the new land for himself, of course after providing the appropriate one-fifth taxation to the King of Spain. To achieve his goal, Velázquez had sent a second expedition commanded by Panfilo de Narváez, a conquistador more loyal to Velázquez than to Cortés, and including an "old crowd" of Caribbean conquistadors. Presumably, they were to aid and strengthen Cortés, but in reality their purpose was to take control from him. Unknown to the Narváez expedition, a slave among the crew carried smallpox. From this expedition, the Spaniards spread smallpox throughout the Yucatan, where they stopped before joining Cortés at Veracruz. Hunyg, the Indian king of the Yucatan, and his eldest son died, as did other native royalty. When Narváez's conquistadors arrived at Veracruz, Cortés won them over, which strengthened his army to slightly under 900 men. It was this small force that occupied Tenochtitlan, the capital of the Aztecs, and imprisoned Montezuma.

On Montezuma's death, his successor as Emperor of Mexico gathered the Aztec forces and led a night attack to drive the conquistadors out of the city. But on that night, smallpox also reached Tenochtitlan. The Emperor of Mexico, many of his family and subjects, and the Aztec troops died of smallpox. As area after area succumbed to infection, many streets were filled with people dead or dying from smallpox, with no method of collecting the bodies. In some places half the population died. Kings and noblemen died as swiftly as farmers and serfs (10):

> Great was the stench of the dead. After our fathers and grandfathers suc-
> cumbed, half the people fled to the fields. The dogs and vultures devoured
> the bodies. The mortality was terrible. Your grandfathers died and with
> them the sons of kings and their brothers and kings men. So it was that we
> became orphans, oh my sons. So we became when we were young. All of us
> were thus. We were born to die.

The disease spread from family to family and from town to town, and famine followed because there were not enough people alive to farm the land.

The havoc wrought by smallpox also brought a morbid state of mind to the Aztecs. They thought the disease supernatural because it preferentially killed them but spared the conquistadors. Most of the Spaniards, having survived to adulthood despite epidemics at home, were immune to smallpox. However, for the Aztecs this exposure was a first-time event. The only interpretation obvious to them was that they were being punished by angry gods. It seemed that the Spanish god was supreme over the Aztec gods, just as the Spanish conquerers came to dominate and obliterate their Aztec foes. Three million Indians, an estimated one-third of the total population in Mexico, was killed at this time by smallpox. The aftermath is not surprising. As the natives docilely accepted commands from the priests and the Spanish authorities, mass conversions to Christianity and to a Spain-like country followed.

This story is by no means the only example of smallpox spreading throughout an isolated, indigenous population with horrendous consequences. By the seventeenth and eighteenth centuries, smallpox was the most devastating disease in the world, in Europe alone killing an estimated 400,000 people each year. One-third of all cases of blindness resulted from smallpox. In 1853, some 80 percent of the native population of Oahu, Hawaii, died when first exposed to smallpox. Even as late as 1903, the South American Cayapo tribe was decimated by smallpox. A single missionary priest, inadvertantly carrying the virus, arrived to work among the 6000 to 8000 Indians. After fifteen years only 500 natives survived.

Rich and poor alike were victims. The use of makeup began among the wealthy who survived smallpox in an attempt to hide their pitted faces. Even the European monarchs were not sequestered from the disease. During this time Queen Mary of England died of smallpox in 1694 at the age of thirty-two. The ruling monarchs Joseph I of Germany, Peter II of Russia, Louis XV of France, and William II of Orange met the same fate.

Battles and the course of history were determined by smallpox infection either purposely or inadvertently. In the war of 1763 between France and England to win North America, smallpox was deliberately spread to Indian tribes under the orders of Sir Geoffrey Amherst, the British Commander-in-Chief in North America (11–14). By Amherst's direction, hostile Indian tribes were provided with blankets contaminated with smallpox: "Could it not be contrived to send the smallpox among those disaffected tribes of Indians? We must, on this occasion, use every stratagem in our power to reduce them" (13).

In response to this request by Amherst, Colonel Henry Bouquet, the ranking British officer for the Pennsylvania frontier replied: "I will try to inoculate the Indians with some blankets that may fall in their hands and take care not to get the disease myself" (14). Captain Ecuyer recorded in his journal that he had given two blankets and a handkerchief from the garrison smallpox hospital to hostile chiefs (indian) with the hope "it will have the desired effects."

British troops were variolated (inoculated with smallpox), but in the early years of the war the rebelling American colonists were not. In 1776 Benedict Arnold led an army of American colonial troops to attack Quebec with the hope of freeing that Canadian city from British rule and adding it to the territory of the thirteen colonies (5,15,16). Of the 10,000 American troops in the attack, 5,500 developed smallpox. One of Arnold's officers wrote, "Those regiments, which had not the smallpox, expected every day to come down with it."

There were not enough tents to shelter even the desperately sick men. The moans of the sick and dying could be heard everywhere. Pits were opened as common graves and filled day after day with corpses as the men died like flies. Governor Jonathan Trumble of Connecticut, who visited the retreating American troops ill with smallpox, wrote, "I did not look into a tent or hut in which I did not find a dead or dying man."

In the same war, the fear of smallpox limited and delayed George Washington's attack on Boston to free it from British control. Washington was concerned about the British use of smallpox as a weapon in the war (1 17):

The information I received that the enemy intended spreading smallpox among us I could not suppose them capable of. I now must give some credit to it as it made its appearance on several of those who last came out of Boston. Every necessary precaution has been taken to prevent its being communicated to the Army, and the General Court will take care that it does not spread throughout the country.

As a consequence of smallpox outbreaks among American colonial troops, in 1777 Washington ordered the entire Continental Army variolated.

On the European continent during the Franco-Prussian War of 1870 to 1871 the Prussian army of over 800,000 soldiers were vaccinated every seven years; these Germans lost fewer than 300 out of 8,360 infected. In contrast, the French army commanders who did not believe in repeated vaccination lost over 23,000 soldiers to smallpox and more than 280,000 became infected.

Smallpox is a severe, contagious, febrile disease characterized by a skin rash with fluid-containing vesicles that enlarge to hold pus (2). What is known about its course and pathogenesis stems from clinical and pathological studies in patients and from detailed laboratory investigations of mice infected with mousepox virus (ectromelia) and rabbits infected with vaccinia virus (18). The smallpox virus gains access to the body by the respiratory route (mouth and nose), where it multiplies first in the mucous membranes and then in nearby lymph nodes. The virus enters the bloodstream and travels to internal organs such as the spleen, lymph nodes, liver, and lungs. The virus then goes through cycles of replication that result in the manufacture of a large viral population. The incubation period from the time of the initial exposure to the onset of disease is approximately twelve days, with a range of seven to seventeen days. Thereafter, the virus invades the blood a second time and this terminates the incubation period, as the infected individual now feels ill. At this acute stage, patients have temperatures of 102°F to 106°F, headache, muscle pain, abdominal pain, vomiting, and prostration. The viruses then spread to the skin, where they multiply in epidermal cells. The characteristic skin eruptions follow in three to four days. Initially the rash is a spot on the skin (macule) then progresses to a raised skin lesion (papule) that fills with fluids (vesicular stage). Finally, the fluids become infected and form pustules in the second week of infection.

The individual with smallpox can transmit the infection at any time from a day before the rash appears until all the lesions have healed and the scabs have fallen off. During the early phase of illness, the virus is transmitted from nasal secretions and cough. When the patient's skin eruptions are fully formed, these lesions themselves also becoming a source of infectious material. Smallpox virus may contaminate clothing, bedding, dust, or other inanimate objects (fomites) and remain infectious for months. It was blankets such as this that General Jeffrey Amherst requested to be given to the Indians of Massachusetts, an early example of premeditated germ warfare.

The terror of smallpox has been constant throughout recorded history. By the turn of the eighteenth century, the disease had become endemic in the major cities of Europe and the British Isles. Nearly one-tenth of all mankind had been killed, crippled or disfigured by smallpox: "No man dared to count his children as his own until after they had had the disease." The nursery rhyme that symbolized both smallpox and the bubonic plague and their usual outcome was: "Ring around the rosie, pocket full of posies, a-tishoo, a-tishoo, all fall down."

It was in this milieu of terror with the deaths of peasants, bourgeoisie, and kings alike that a way of preventing smallpox was sought. Variolation, the transfer of smallpox as an inoculum into susceptible individuals, is believed to have occurred in China as early as the first century. Documents record its practice in the Sung Dynasty from 960 to 1280. Variolation consisted of obtaining dried smallpox scabs, converting them into a powder, and inhaling the substance through the nose. From China to India the technique of variolation spread, reaching Persia and Turkey. The most common alternative to this technique of variolation was to remove the thick liquid from the small-pox pustule and rub it into a needle scratch made on the arm.

The Royal Society of London was first informed of the practice of vario-lation around 1700 and began collecting data on the procedure during the first decade of the eighteenth century, primarily from one of its members, the physician Emanuel Timoni (19). Dr. Timoni had received his medical degree from the University of Padua and from Oxford. He later served as the physi-cian to the British Ambassador's family in Constantinople. There he observed variolation and documented the procedure for the Royal Society. His reports detailed withdrawal of the fluid from a pustule of a patient with uncompli-cated smallpox on day twelve or thirteen of illness, then pressing the fluid into a clean glass container and transferring this material onto fresh cuts made by a needle through the fleshy part of a recipients' arm. Lady Mary Montagu, wife of the British Ambassador to Turkey, observed this procedure done in 1718.

As a great beauty, Lady Montagu had a horrifying experience with small-pox when, at the age of twenty-six, she became infected. Although she recov-ered, her face was permanently disfigured. Her brother was not as lucky; he died of the disease. Fearing a smallpox attack on her six-year-old son, she had him variolated during her husband's absence from Constantinople, presum-ably because he objected to the procedure. But Lord Montagu was not alone in his reluctance toward variolation. The British Embassy Chaplain raged that variolation was un-Christian and could succeed only in infidels. However, the variolation done in spite of his fierce and sustained opposition was super-vised by Dr. Timoni and performed by Dr. Maitland, the Scottish Embassy surgeon. The procedure was a success and Lady Montagu's son resisted small-pox infection.

Lady Montagu later informed her friend, Carolene of Anspach, the Princess of Wales and later the Queen of England during George II's reign, of the variolation procedure. Lady Montagu described vividly its effectiveness in the many cases that she had seen, particularly her son. In 1721, during an out-break of smallpox in London, the Princess of Wales asked Dr. Maitland to var-iolate her three-year-old daughter. Shortly thereafter, the Prince and Princess of Wales, along with members of the Royal Society, had Dr. Maitland vario-late six condemned prisoners at Newgate. The prisoners' reward for undergo-ing variolation was freedom if they survived the procedure and resisted an active exposure to smallpox. Witnessed by over twenty-five members of the Royal Society and reported publicly by newspapers, variolation showed a dra-matic protective effect. One of the three women variolated, Elizabeth Harri-son, later went to Hertford during a smallpox epidemic. There she failed to develop the disease despite nursing a hospitalized patient with active smallpox and lying in bed with a child of six, who had smallpox for six weeks. This and other accounts of successful variolation were published by Maitland in a book dedicated to the Prince and Princess of Wales. Maitland later traveled to the European continent to variolate Prince Frederick of Hanover. Thereafter physicians came from all parts of Europe to learn the procedure, which was supervised by the Royal Society and sponsored by the Prince and Princess of Wales. The end result was that variolation protected many recipients exposed to smallpox later in life, although its use was associated with a 2 percent death rate.

Variolation in the United States began along an independent path. In 1706, the Reverend Cotton Mather of Boston heard about variolation as practiced in Africa from his African slave. After acquiring additional information from slave traders, Mather obtained and read Dr. Timoni's article (19) describing variolation as published in *Philosophical Transactions*. Mather then began actively seeking physicians in Boston to perform variolation as a defense against the attacks of smallpox that frequently cycled through the community. One physician, Zabdiel Boylston, of Brookline, Massachusetts, successfully variolated his six-year-old son, his thirty-year-old slave, and the slave's two-year-old son. Boylston reported these results in the *Boston Gazette* on the July 17, 1721, along with those from the successful variolation of seven other persons. By 1722 he had variolated 242 patients, six of whom died. His data indicated a mortality rate of 2.5 percent in those variolated as compared with the ordinarily 15 to 20 percent dead during most smallpox epidemics. It was this report detailing the experience of Boylston, coupled with deaths of soldiers in his army from smallpox, that led George Washington to variolate troops of the Continental Army. The popularity of variolation continued until Edward Jenner provided the safer alternative of vaccination in 1798. Louis Pasteur, the great microbiologist who in 1879 attenuated fowl cholera bacteria by lengthening its passage in culture and who experimentally worked out the conditions for attenuation of bacteria and viruses, adopted the word "vaccine" to describe the generalized group of immunizing products. He chose the word in recognition of Jenner's work on the cowpox (*vacca*, Latin for cow) vaccine and vaccination procedure. With use of the most attenuated cowpox virus vaccines instead of variolation with smallpox virus, the incidence of death was reduced from two to three per hundred to one per 100,000 to one per million.

Edward Jenner, an eighteenth-century country physician in the market town of Berkeley in Gloucestershire, England, had observed that cowmaids in his area had fair and almost perfect complexions when compared with the disfiguring pockmarks of villagers infected with smallpox:

Where are you going, my pretty maid
I'm going a-milking, sir, she said
May I go with you, my pretty maid
You're kindly welcome, sir, she said
What is your father, my pretty maid
My father's a farmer, sir, she said
What is your fortune, my pretty maid
My face is my fortune, sir, she said.

He was aware that cowmaids who had been exposed to the pox infection of cows (cowpox) did not develop smallpox. In 1796 he obtained a cowpox vesicle, induced by cowpox, from the hand of his patient Sarah Nilmes and transferred it to the skin of a young lad, James Phipps. Later, when Phipps was exposed to and even inoculated with smallpox, he resisted smallpox infection. These and similar observations convinced Jenner of the feasibility and the benefits of vaccinating susceptible individuals with cowpox (current vaccine is called vaccinia) as a preventive therapy against the development of smallpox. Jenner eventually provided a detailed protocol for vaccination accompanied by illustrations of the procedure and the expected findings (20). Yet, Jenner was not the first to vaccinate against smallpox. Benjamin Jesty, a farmer and cattle breeder in Dorchester, vaccinated his wife and two sons with materials taken directly from cowpox

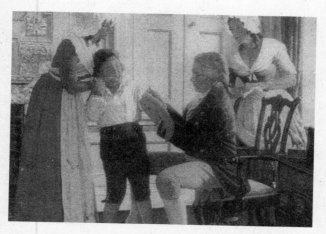

Figure 4.4 The first vaccination is depicted in this painting. Edward Jenner is seen vaccinating eight-year-old James Phipps with vesicle fluid taken from the cowpox lesion on the hand of milkmaid Sarah Nilmes. Courtesy of the Wellcome Trust.

lesions on the udder of a cow from the herd of his neighbor, Mr. Elford. Jesty had been aware of the beneficial effect of using cowpox to protect against smallpox. Previously he had noticed that two of his servant girls who had cowpox showed solid resistance to smallpox upon repeated exposure to the disease. He had known of other similar instances from reports of his neighbors. No doubt other laymen also performed similar prophylactic measures using materials obtained directly from infected cows. In 1764, thirty-two years before Jenner inoculated James Phipps with cowpox, Angelo Gatti published *Reflexions on Variolation*, which described its benefits and the nature of smallpox infection. He even discussed the need to find a means of attenuating the smallpox virus so as to diminish the morbidity and mortality it caused.

In addition to his medical practice, Jenner was a keen naturalist. He collected fossils and biological specimens for study, and investigated the breeding of toads and eels, and when Joseph Banks returned from Captain Cook's circumnavigation of the Pacific in 1771, he approached Jenner for assistance in the classification of botanical materials he collected. Jenner was the first to describe cuckoo hatchlings ejecting the other eggs from the nest and nestling of the foster parents. On the basis of these studies and publication of *The Natural History of the Cuckoo* he became a Fellow of the British Royal Society. Although Jenner had published in the *Royal Society Journal*, he was refused the opportunity either to present or publish his observations about smallpox. This

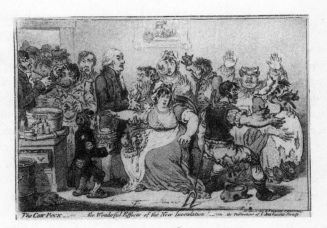

*Figure 4.5 Not all thought the procedure of vaccination to be wonderful.
Painting by the anti-vaccinationist James Gillnay in 1802 shows
vaccinated persons with parts of cows growing out of their arms and bodies.
Courtesy of the Wellcome Trust.*

rejection by the Royal Society was accompanied by the message that "he was in variance with established knowledge" and that "he had better not promulgate such a wild idea if he valued his reputation."

Luckily for mankind, Jenner disregarded the rebuff from this learned and prominent society and published his results at his own expense two years later. Jenner's pamphlet, *An Inquiry into the Causes and Effects of the Variolae Vaccinae, a Disease Discovered in Some of the Western Counties of England, Particularly Gloucestershire and Known by the Name of Cowpox*, contained careful descriptions of twenty patients whose lasting immunity to smallpox followed vaccination with cowpox. The importance of this singular contribution was recognized by many, but not all, of his contemporaries. Opponents argued that vaccination was a revolting practice, that to infect a healthy person with repugnant material from an animal was an outrage, that vaccinated victims sprouted horns and looked like cows, and that one was interfering with God's way, since vaccination was not mentioned in the Bible. This opposition was mounted by those in the medical and business professions as well as by religious leaders. Even the poet Lord Byron classified cowpox as a passing fancy.

> Now look around, and turn each trifling page,
> survey the precious works that please the age;
> what varied wonders tempt us as they pass!
> The cowpox, tractors, galvanism, and gas in turn appears

But Jenner weathered these blows; his pamphlet was read and his technique rapidly applied in areas of Britain, the European continent, as well as North and South America. Jenner himself received letters of gratitude from admirers worldwide. For example, in 1806, President Thomas Jefferson wrote to congratulate Jenner on his great achievement. "Yours is the comfortable reflection that mankind can never forget that you have lived. Future nations will know by history only that the loathsome smallpox had existed and by you has been extirpated." Napoleon, who was at the time at war with Britain, released English prisoners of war and permitted English citizens to return home upon the request of Jenner. Napoleon remarked that he could not "refuse anything to such a great benefactor of mankind." The Chiefs of the Five Nations of the North American Indians sent a wampum belt with a letter of thanks to Jenner in 1807. Their people had suffered grievously from smallpox, both inadvertently as passed by infected Europeans and directly by deliberate introduction of blankets contaminated with smallpox. The results were the killings of hundreds of thousands of their tribe members. Their letter said, "Brother: Our

Father has delivered to us the book you sent to instruct us how to use the discovery which the Great Spirit made to you whereby the smallpox, that fatal enemy of our tribe, may be driven from the earth. . . . We sent with this a belt and a string of wampum in token of our appreciation of your precious gift." Of his many awards, Jenner especially valued the belt. He wore it with pride on ceremonial occasions. In Britain he received financial rewards of £10,000 and £20,000 in 1802 and 1807, respectively. Jenner was appointed Physician Extraordinary to his majesty, King George IV.

Yet there was overt and noisy controversy over vaccination. One example is the case of Benjamin Waterhouse and James Smith in the United States (21,22). Benjamin Waterhouse was appointed Professor of Theory and Practice of Physics at the newly established Harvard Medical School in 1783 after returning to Boston from several years of study abroad. For eight years he had studied at the best medical schools of that time, the University of Edinburgh, Scotland, and the University of Leiden, Holland. After receiving his medical degree from the University of Leiden, he stayed at the university for an additional session and boarded with John Adams, the American minister. Adams would later become the second President of the United States. Waterhouse arrived at Harvard in 1783. From friends in England he later received a copy of Jenner's publication in 1799. Thereafter, Waterhouse devoted his energies to advocating the use of cowpox to vaccinate against smallpox, rather than using variolation. Waterhouse received a glass vial containing cowpox directly from Jenner. He used it to vaccinate his son and others. Those vaccinated resisted infection when exposed to natural smallpox or when variolated with smallpox. However, many other physicians in the Boston area were opposed to vaccination. A coalition of physicians from Harvard and the Boston community petitioned the Boston Board of Health in 1802 to set up and conduct a public test of the new vaccine. Although it may not have been their intent, this investigation clearly proved the superiority of vaccination over variolation. The board then urged doctors to accept the principle of vaccination. Subsequently Waterhouse wrote to Thomas Jefferson and sent him his pamphlet on "A Prospect of Eliminating Smallpox." Jefferson wrote back, "Every friend of humanity must look with pleasure at this discovery, by which one more evil is withdrawn from the condition of man; and most contemplate the possibility that future improvements and discoveries may still more and more lessen the catalogue of the evils."

Jefferson himself became actively involved in the fight to vaccinate (23,24). Through his efforts, vaccine material received from Waterhouse was distributed to Jefferson's native Virginia, then to Pennsylvania and numerous areas within the south. Jefferson also sent Jenner's vaccine with Meriwether Lewis and William Clark on their journey to explore the Louisiana Purchase and find passage to the Pacific Ocean. He instructed Lewis on its use and requested it be brought to the frontier and Indians (25). Finally, James Madison, the fourth President of the United States, who was familiar with both Jefferson's and Waterhouse's activities, signed legislation, the first of its kind, to encourage vaccination.

To put this critical medical therapy into practice, Dr. James Smith of Maryland was appointed as the federal agent for the distribution of the vaccine. However, the winds still blew strongly against the use of vaccination. Politically, Waterhouse was a religious Quaker and, as such, a pacifist. Despite its popularity, he had objected to the Revolutionary War. To avoid entanglement in the war he traveled to and lived in Britain in the early part of 1775. Further, he was born in Rhode Island and was considered an outsider to many in the Boston community. Finally, his political sympathies were with Thomas Jefferson and his style of government, a Populist democracy. By contrast to Waterhouse, the Boston elite supported Federalism and considered Jefferson immoral. As so often repeated in history, political power overcame good sense. A coalition of physicians at Harvard and throughout Boston, in concert with church leaders, arranged the dismissal of Waterhouse from his chair at the Harvard Medical School in 1812. Accordingly, the changing political climate in Washington in the 1820s led to repeal of the vaccine law followed by the dismissal of James Smith from his office in 1822. The result was that by 1840, epidemics of smallpox and deaths that followed once again increased in the United States.

Jenner and Jefferson expressed the hope in the early nineteenth century that smallpox might someday be eliminated. However, it was over 150 years after Jenner proved the effectiveness of vaccination that the first serious proposal to undertake smallpox eradication appeared. In 1950, the Pan-American Sanitary Organization made the commitment to conquer smallpox throughout the Americas. A program of mass vaccinations eliminated smallpox by the 1970s from all countries in the Americas except for Argentina, Brazil, Colombia, and Ecuador, where the number of cases was markedly reduced.

With governments around the world conducting vaccination programs, outbreaks of smallpox came under control in many but not all countries. In 1953, Dr. Brock Chisholm, the first Director General of the World Health Organization (WHO), proposed that smallpox eradication be undertaken as a global effort, and he challenged member states of WHO to join this crusade (2,26–28). However, the initial response of the World Health Assembly was not encouraging. Representatives of virtually every industrialized country, including the United States, argued that such a program was too complicated, too vast. So Chisholm's proposal was dropped (2). In fairness, at this time, WHO was preoccupied with a costly program to eradicate malaria, which occupied the majority of its efforts and budget. Unfortunately, this program turned out to be disappointing, yet during this period smallpox was successfully eliminated from several more countries, including China. Five years later the Vice Minister of Health of the Soviet Union, Victor Zhadnov, proposed a ten-year program for the eradication of smallpox. Reasoning that the USSR had eradicated smallpox throughout its vast and ethnically heterogeneous country, he argued that there was no reason why other countries around the world could not do likewise. With the prodding of Zhadnov and others, the WHO Assembly finally did vote to accept the program, in principle, but unrealistically delegated only $100,000 of its budget. This lack of funding effectively defeated the proposal. At this time even the influential and prominent microbiologist Rene Dubos, like Lord Byron 150 years earlier, referred to smallpox eradication as a passing fancy: "Make it probably useless to discuss the theoretical flaws and technical difficulties of eradication programs, because more earthly factors will certainly bring them soon to a gentle and silent death. . . . Eradication programs will eventually become a curiosity item on library shelves, just as have all social utopias."

Nevertheless, the fight for eradication did not stop. In 1966, the WHO Director General, Marcelino Candau, proposed a budget of $2.4 million for smallpox eradication. Incredibly, almost every industrialized country again protested the size of the budget, and most expressed doubts about the wisdom of the program. Thus discovery by Jenner that would lead to one of the major accomplishments of mankind became implemented by a margin of only two votes. Under the direction of D. A. Henderson and his colleagues, WHO directed considerable effort toward the eradication of smallpox.

Donald Ainslie Henderson was born in Lakewood, Ohio, in 1928. He received his medical training at the University of Rochester and public health training at Johns Hopkins. He worked in the area of disease surveillance at the Centers for Disease Control until assuming the position of Chief Medical Officer for the Smallpox Eradication Program of the WHO in 1966. He directed that program until the eradication of smallpox. Henderson used two principal strategies. First, international vaccine testing centers were developed to ensure that all vaccines met the standards of safety and effectiveness. This guaranteed that only active vaccine would be used. Second, reducing the number of smallpox cases to zero became the established goal rather than documenting the number of vaccine doses given. With this goal, effective surveillance teams were set up to both report and contain outbreaks of smallpox.

In the early years of the program, it became clear that the number of small-pox cases was underreported and that only 10 percent of vaccines being pro-duced or provided met the accepted international standards. Subsequently, with more accurate surveillance and reporting, with the use of only those vaccines approved by the international vaccine testing centers, and with a program for vigorous vaccination of peoples in Africa and Asia, by 1970 smallpox was eliminated from twenty countries of Western and Central Africa. In 1971, smallpox was eliminated from Brazil, in 1972 from Indonesia, in 1975 from the entire Asian continent, in 1976 from Ethiopia, and in 1977 the last case was reported in Somalia. Thus by 1980, 184 years after Edward Jenner inoculated James Phipps and 182 years after he published *An Inquiry into the Causes and Effects of the Variolae Vaccinae* . . . the World Health Assembly announced worldwide eradication of smallpox. This singular event is one of the greatest accomplishments undertaken and performed for the benefit of mankind anywhere or at any time.

The microbe hunters who accomplished this deed are many, but can be placed into two groups. First and unquestionably was Edward Jenner, his work, perseverence, and influence. Second is the large group of dedicated health care workers who traveled to the distant corners of the earth to track cases of smallpox and to vaccinate all peoples on the globe. This group was lead by D. A. Henderson. Henderson reflects the best qualities of many in the long line of public health officers in the United States and throughout the world who have devoted their energies both scientifically and politically toward the control and elimination of infectious diseases.

The success of the Smallpox Eradication Program indicates clearly that other viruses with characteristics similar to smallpox—that is, whose natural host is man, which have no animal intermediate, and do not cause persistent infection—such as measles and poliomyelitis, can and should be eradicated. Scientific research has provided the tools; all that remains is the political and economic willpower and desire to do so. Thus smallpox, one of the viruses most intently studied by newly emerging practitioners of medicine, and a killer of millions of people, is becoming no more than a curiosity, likely be removed from the teaching curriculum of medical schools. There are plans to eliminate all stocks of smallpox within the next several years, thus making the virus the first species purposely eliminated from this planet.

CHAPTER 5

YELLOW FEVER

Yellow fever, also called yellow jack or the yellow plague, became one of the most feared diseases throughout the Americas in the nineteenth century. This endemic disease of West Africa traveled to the New World and elsewhere aboard trading ships with their cargoes of slaves. These African blacks, although easily infected, nevertheless withstood the effects so that fewer died from the infection than did Caucasians, American Indians, or Asians. Ironically, as smallpox and measles devastated natives along the Caribbean coast and islands, growing numbers of African slaves were brought to replace those plantation laborers. When the value of Africans over natives became apparent, by virtue of the blacks' resistance to yellow fever, the importation of these Africans increased still further (1,2).

Because it was so lethal for susceptible humans, yellow fever actually disrupted exploration into the Caribbean. In fact, American expansion became possible only after a team led by Walter Reed arrived in Cuba to combat the disease and prove it was transmitted by the *Aedes aegypti* mosquito. In 1901, a campaign was launched to eliminate yellow fever from Havana by attacking mosquito breeding places, a plan that proved effective. Finally, in 1937, a successful vaccine was developed.

From the sixteenth to the early twentieth century, yellow fever remained a dread and mysterious disease of unknown cause. Not even imagined hundreds of years ago was that the *Aedes aegypti* mosquito dwelling in the jungles of West Africa carried the yellow fever virus as part of a monkey-to-mosquito cycle. When humans penetrated into areas traveled by infected monkeys, the disease was then transmitted via infected female mosquitos. The insects live only about 70 to 160 days, although maximal survival of 225 days has been reported, and the flight range of the insect is less than 300 meters. The mosquito lays its eggs in still water, a breeding habitat that includes water–filled cans, bottles, urns, and crevices (3,4). Consequently, the mosquito is an excellent traveler on boats and migrated successfully from West Africa to the Caribbean by that means. Because yellow fever was unknown in pre-Columbian America, and Native Americans showed the same susceptibility as the colonists, it is safe to assume that the disease arrived here along with trans-oceanic shipping (5,6). The disease was first recorded in 1648 in the Yucatan and Havana as an abrupt and short-lived fever lasting three to four days followed by a brief remission stage and then a second feverish stage when jaundice or yellowing appeared. Because liver injury associated with infection disrupted normal clotting of blood, many patients bled from nose and gums and frequently vomited blood (black vomit). Most of these victims died within eight days of the fever's reappearance.

As trade by ocean-going vessels continued, yellow fever struck Brazil in 1686, Martinique in 1690, Cadiz, Spain, in 1730, and later Marseilles, France, and the port of Swansea (1878) in Wales. Knowing that victims of yellow fever must be isolated from other patients and the general population, the staff of Greenwich Hospital in England dressed the segregated patients in jackets with yellow patches to forewarn others about the contagion. They were nicknamed "Yellow Jackets," and a yellow-colored flag that flew over the quarantined area was referred to as the "Yellow Jack."

Outbreaks in North American port cities included those in New York and Philadelphia. In the Philadelphia epidemic of 1793, some 4,044 individuals (over 10%) among the city's population of less than 40,000 perished in four months (7–10). Most likely the source was mosquitos in water barrels aboard ships that transported French refugees fleeing the yellow fever scourge of 1792–9 in Santo Domingo, Haiti, and the West Indies (7,8,10).

In 1793 Philadelphia was America's capital. George Washington, John

Adams, Thomas Jefferson, Alexander Hamilton, and John Knox witnessed the yellow fever plague and watched as it shut down the United States government. In July, one ship, then another, then fleets flocked in from Santo Domingo and the West Indies discharging hordes of refugees, white and black. Hungry and sickly, they poured into Philadelphia bringing news of the ongoing revolution in the islands. They told of the carnage, slaughter, destruction of plantations, and pestilent fever raging throughout the islands, and the agony of fevers on board the ships.

During that summer heavy rains descended on Philadelphia and produced a great increase of mosquitos, a nuisance to those living in the city. Denny's Lodging House in North Water Street was a favorite place of residence for sailors and new arrivals, of which several from Santo Domingo and the other Caribbean islands found their way (10). Two French sailors had taken a room at Denny's, and one was soon stricken with fever and died. Several days later the second sailor died. Two other boarders at Denny's died shortly therefter, and many others in the city became feverish and died. The fever had begun to spread. Stories told of a victim's "wretched state without a pulse, with cold clammy hands and his face a yellow color," of his "great distress, feverish, with yellow color on his skin, nauseated, throwing-up black vomit and given to nose-bleeds."

When a quarantine was put into effect but failed to stop the yellow fever, the authorities decided that the disease was not imported. Instead, they asserted that local conditions of rotting coffee by the wharf and garbage in the streets caused putrid air that transmitted the disease (10,11). Dr. Benjamin Rush, one of the leading physicians of the time advised everyone who could to leave the city, to travel into the countryside where the air was clear (11): "There is only one way to prevent the disease—fly from it."

Philadelphia had suffered a previous yellow fever plague in 1762, when a hundred had died, but now thousands were dying. Thomas Jefferson wrote from Philadelphia to James Madison in Virginia, telling about the fever, how everyone who could was fleeing and how one of every three stricken had died. Alexander Hamilton, the Secretary of the Treasury, came down with the fever. He left town, but when he was refused entry to New York City, he turned to upstate New York, to the home of his wife's father in Green Bush near Albany. There he and his wife were obliged to stay under armed guard until their clothing and baggage had been burned, their servants and carriage disinfected.

Clerks in departments of the federal government could not be kept at their desks. In the Treasury Department, six clerks got yellow fever and five others fled to New York; three sickened in the post office and seven officers in the customs service. Government papers were locked up in closed houses when the clerks left. By September, the American government came to a standstill. George Washington left for Mount Vernon:

It was my wish to continue there longer—but as Mrs. Washington was unwilling to leave me surrounded by the malignant fever—I could not think of hazarding her and the children any longer by my continuance in the city—the house in which we lived being, in a manner, blockaded by the disorder and was becoming every day more and more fatal.

Washington recommended removing the clerks and the entire War Office out of Philadelphia. Washington, Jefferson, Hamilton, and Secretary of War Knox all left.

Philip Freneau wrote in 1793 in Philadelphia:

PESTILENCE
Written During the Prevalence of a Yellow Fever

Hot, dry winds forever blowing,
Dead men to the grave-yards going:
    Constant hearses,
    Funeral verses;
Oh! what plagues—there is no knowing!
Priests retreating from their pulpits!—
Some in hot, and some in cold fits
    In bad temper,
    Off they scamper,
Leaving us—unhappy culprits!
Doctors raving and disputing,
Death's pale army still recruiting—
    What a pother
    One with t'other!
Some a-writing, some a-shooting.
Nature's poisons here collected,
Water, earth, and air infected—
    O, what pity,
    Such a city,
Was in such a place erected!

The cause of yellow fever, a virus, would not be discovered until 100 years later in Cuba, and the route of transmission (mosquito as the vector) would not be implicated until eight years after that discovery. These plagues in New York and Philadelphia were limited primarily to the summer, because *Aedes aegypti* mosquitos prefer warm, tropical climates and do not survive in the frost. So it was in the tropical climates in and around the Caribbean, Central and Latin America, and the southern United States that the mosquito flourished and caused repeated epidemics. These outbreaks could be dramatic, as on the island of Santo Domingo, where in three months of 1793 over 44 percent of British soldiers forming the 41st Foot Regiment and 23rd Guard died. Refugees from such attacks who incubated the virus as they fled to cities of North America and Europe continued to spread the disease when they came in contact with the carrier mosquitos.

Most black Africans and their descendants respond to yellow fever infection with mild to moderate symptoms such as headache, fever, nausea, and vomiting, and then recover in a few days. This outcome reflects the long relationship between the virus and its indigenous hosts, who through generations of exposure to the virus have evolved resistance. In some victims, the fever is more pronounced, rising to 104°F, along with generalized joint pains and bleeding. Still, even these patients recover within a few days. In contrast, among Caucasians and American Indians, the disease assumes epidemic proportions and unfolds in a severe, three-stage course. During the first stage, an infection with fever of 102°F to 105°F lasts three to four days, during which the patient is infectious. Headache, back and muscle pain, nausea, and vomiting are severe. Thereafter, a remission stage without fever, or period of calm ensues, sometimes lasting for just a few hours as the temperature falls to 99°F–100°F, the headache disappears, and the patient feels better. Then the third stage occurs. The temperature rapidly rises again, and symptoms present in the first stage recur but in more severe form, as the patient becomes increasingly agitated and anxious. Liver, heart, and/or renal failure follow, which leads to delirium. Jaundice, or yellowing of the skin, develops at about the fourth or fifth day during this third stage of disease. Within six to seven days, death frequently follows. Those who survive remain ill, usually for another seventeen to thirty days. Thereafter, recovery is slow and marked by intense fatigue.

Imagine this setting at a time when Napoleon had plans for an American empire. His base was French-controlled areas in the Caribbean, parts of Central America, Mexico, New Orleans, and the North American Midwest extending to Canada. Haiti, colonized by the French, was run by African labor. In 1801, a rebellion of this work force headed by the black leader Toussaint Louverture caused Napoleon to counter with a military expedition under his brother-in-law, General LeClerc (12). But within a few months

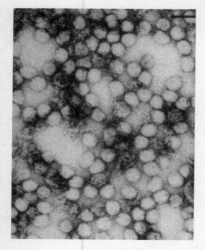

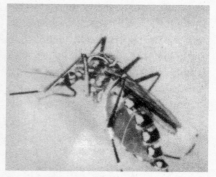

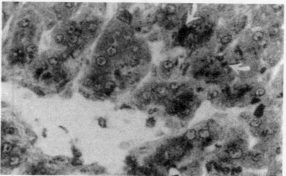

Figure 5.1 Photomicrograph of the morphology of the yellow fever virus
(top left) *and the vector, the* Aedes aegypti *mosquito* (top right). *The
virion particles are morphologically indistinct except that they are compact
and relatively homogeneous in size. Bar, 100 nm. Electron micrograph
from E. L. Palmer and M. L. Martin,* An Atlas of Mammalian Viruses
(1982), courtesy of CRC Press, Inc. (bottom). *Liver destruction of a
patient who died from yellow fever virus infection. The arrows point to
deposits of yellow fever virus antigen. This picture courtesy of* Fields'
Virology *(Philadelphia: Lippincott-Raven, 1996).*

after this force arrived in Santo Domingo, yellow fever destroyed over 27,000
of the veteran French troops, including LeClerc, leaving but few survivors.
The disease had little effect on the black troops under Louverture. The results
of this French defeat were twofold. First, Haiti gained its freedom from

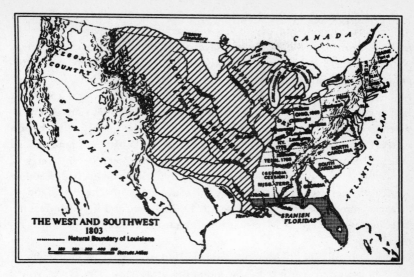

Figure 5.2 The effect of yellow fever on history is shown by the addition of the Louisiana Territory to the United States. Devastation of Napoleon's troops in Haiti from yellow fever and the need to focus his resources on the Egyptian campaign and wars against England led to the sale of this territory to the United States government in 1803 under the direction of Thomas Jefferson.

France. Second, Napoleon's ambitions in the New World dissolved. Disenchanted with his American venture, he decided to sell the Louisiana Territory to the United States (12). This act changed the destiny of the New World, since removal of the French influence allowed American growth westward into new channels, and eliminated potential agitation between the two countries over land that America would have fought to acquire. Napoleon then redirected his empire building toward new efforts on Malta and in Egypt.

Unlike the sporadic record-keeping for early smallpox and measles epidemics, the events of yellow fever epidemics in the nineteenth century are relatively clear because of the careful documentation and the rapid communication available. The spread of yellow fever and the devastation and fear it brought were portrayed by word of mouth and newspapers as this disease rampaged along the Mississippi and into Memphis, Tennessee, in the dark year of 1878. Just before the American Civil War in 1861, Memphis had a population of 22,000, which rose to 48,000 by 1878. In a few months, this vibrant and expanding town found its population reduced by over one-half from the devastation and deaths from yellow fever (13, 14).

According to eyewitnesses of that time, Memphis was the hub of one of the world's major cotton-producing regions. It was located on America's major trade routes—the Mississippi River and three railroad lines. Its citizens were old-stock Southern whites, newly freed African Americans, and immigrants mainly from Ireland but also from Germany, France, Italy, and China. None living in Memphis at that time or elsewhere in the world knew that insects could transmit disease. But the *Aedes aegypti* mosquito lurked everywhere up and down the Mississippi River. All that was missing was a person whose blood contained the yellow fever virus. Once the mosquitos bit an infected human and ingested that infected blood, the insects became carriers, or vectors, of the disease whose subsequent bites infected every susceptible individual contacted. Thus the spread of disease began. The event and its progress were recorded in the Memphis *Daily Appeal*, and by J. M. Keating, its editor, who stayed in Memphis throughout the ordeal and published his recollections (15).

Mrs. Kate Bionda of Memphis and her husband ran a small restaurant/snack house located in Front Row along the great Mississippi River, where their main trade was catering food and drink to riverboat men. Mosquitoes were nuisances, especially during this summer of 1878. In late July, cases of yellow fever were noted in New Orleans. The *Daily Appeal* reported on July 24th:

We learn from New Orleans that 24 people have died of yellow fever there in the past few days. We need not fear in Memphis. We were never in as good a condition from the sanitary point of view. Our streets and alleys were never as clean, and strict attention is now being paid to the enforcement of sanitary regulations on private premises. Nothing in our atmosphere invites that dread disease. There are no grounds for alarm on the part of our people. The yellow fever is not endogenous to our latitude and unless imported there is no reason to fear it. It cannot be imported as long as our sanitary laws are enforced.

Nevertheless, public apprehension increased on August sixth when the press carried news of a New Orleans steamboat hand's death from yellow fever at the quarantine hospital on President's Island. The victim, William Warren, had slipped into Memphis, stopped at the Bionda's restaurant on the night of August 1 and became sick on August 2. He was admitted to the city hospital, where his illness was diagnosed as yellow fever, and then moved to the quarantine hospital where he died on August 5. A few days later, Mrs. Bionda, age thirty-four, became ill, and she died on August 13. On the basis of her clinical course including jaundice, her physician diagnosed her condition as the first case of yellow fever in Memphis in 1878.

Yellow fever was no stranger to people living along the Mississippi River or in the Mississippi valley. But, as yet, Memphis had not suffered anything like the great New Orleans epidemic of 1853 that killed 9000 persons. However, yellow fever had visited Memphis before—killing 75 people in 1855, 250 in 1867, and 2000 in 1873—so the citizenry knew that the attacks were growing worse as the city grew. Even so, the greatest fear of yellow fever came from the unknown—how it came about, how it spread. Yellow fever was as mysterious to nineteenth century people everywhere, including Memphis, as were the great plagues of the Middle Ages to its populations. What was known about yellow fever was that it could spread relatively easily from city to city and that quarantine of incoming goods or people from yellow fever-infected areas limited or prevented the spread of disease.

It is believed that the practice of quarantine began in 1374, first in the Venetian Republic and then in Milan (16). Quarantine was derived from the Italian word *quaranta*, or forty days, and indicated the time allotted for isolation. Its purpose then, as now, was to isolate people from infected places, especially during the bubonic plague. The penalty for breaking of quarantine was frequently death. In 1383, Marseilles practiced quarantines regularly, setting a limit of forty days, and by the fifteenth century most European countries had detention stations to confine the infected.

But yellow fever, unlike other plagues, smallpox, or measles, did not spread from person to person by contact. Yet the authorities understood that people fleeing from a community where yellow fever struck could in some unexplained way spread the disease to the place where they sought asylum. Thus, cities attempted to prevent entry by escapees from disease centers and prohibited their inhabitants from entering affected areas.

The tracking of yellow fever began in late spring and early summer of 1878 when the disease was reported in the West Indies, an area involved in trade with cities along the Mississippi River. The possibility of another epidemic like the one of 1873 grew in the minds of some of the Memphis populace, especially physicians and health board members, who argued vigorously for quarantine measures before the city council. But business interests on the council rejected quarantine for fear of disrupting their lucrative trade. As a result, the president of the Board of Health, Dr. R. W. Mitchell, resigned in protest. The quarantine debate continued as yellow fever spread closer, first reported in cities along the West Indies and then by July 26 in New Orleans roughly 500 miles away from Memphis. With outbreaks in New Orleans on July 26, and in Vicksburg, only 240 miles away, on July 27, Memphis finally established quarantine stations for goods and people from those cities. But would quarantine or any man-made edicts work? Fear and rumor spread through Memphis and multiplied when, on August 5, a man taken from a riverboat and hospitalized in Memphis was diagnosed as having yellow fever. By August 9 yellow fever was on the march as people in the city of Grenada, just ninety miles south of Memphis, reported attacks. The news spread quickly by word of mouth. Memphis newspapers tried to calm an increasingly agitated public:

> The public may rely upon it that whenever yellow fever shows itself, as is not likely, the Board of Health through the press of the city, will promptly report it. Keep cool! Avoid patent medicines and bad whiskey! Go about your business as usual; be cheerful and laugh as much as possible (15,17).

The advice was not easy to take. Although some calm returned to the city, residents began to leave Memphis, and others considered the possibility of doing so or began making preparations, just in case. By this time Mrs. Bionda was dying from yellow fever. On August 14, the day after she died, fifty-five additional cases were announced; by August15 and 16 a full panic was under way. By foot, by railroad, by horse, by wagon, thousands of people began to leave: "On any road leading out of Memphis was a procession of wagons piled high with beds, trunks, small furniture, carrying also women and children. Beside walked men, some riotous, with the wild excitement, others moody and silent from anxiety and dread" (18).

Railroad companies attached extra cars, but these were not enough for all the people trying to push inside. Civic institutions collapsed. As city councilmen and aldermen fled, the city council was unable to assemble a quorum. One-third of the police force deserted. The fear of refugees evacuating Memphis mimicked the emotions of refugees fleeing advancing German armies during the Second World War in Europe. They ran from the unknown, from death. By four days after Mrs. Bionda's death, over half the population of Memphis, more than 25,000 people, had fled to small towns along the Mississippi River, to Virginia, East Tennessee, St. Louis, Cincinnati, Louisville, and elsewhere.

Bitter experiences met some of these refugees. Towns along their route established quarantines against those coming from Memphis. Citizens enforced barricades with rifles and shotguns. Officials in Little Rock, Arkansas, refused to let railroad trains from Memphis near their city. Others fleeing on riverboats, like the steamship *John D. Porter*, traveled up the Mississippi but were forced to stay on board for two months as port after port refused them permission to land, like the cursed *Flying Dutchman*, which was condemned to roam the seas eternally.

Many of the refugees did carry yellow fever and entered areas where the *Aedes aegypti* mosquito lived, thereby continuing the spread of disease along the Mississippi. Over 100 people fleeing from Memphis died outside the city. But what about the 20,000 who remained in Memphis? Of these citizens, roughly 14,000 were African Americans and 6,000 were whites (18). Terror-stricken, they awaited their unknown fate, aware that the mysterious disease would rage until the frost came in late October. The question was could they stay alive for the remaining forty-five or so days?

The epidemic struck with frightening swiftness and severity. Within a week of Kate Bionda's death, thousands were sick. As recorded by a minister in attendance, "weeks of suffering before us . . . numbers dying for want of attention which we are powerless to give. . . . God help us." At least 200 people died per day through the first half of September. Eleven weeks after the initial case, there were 17,000 cases, 5,000 of which were fatal (18).

During these harrowing weeks, the city was tomb-like. Few ventured into the street, all commercial activity stopped. Robert Blakeslee, a New Yorker who came to Memphis by train to help fight the disease, described for the *New York Herald* the following interview on walking from the railroad depot:

> The city was almost deserted. . . . We had not gone far, however, before the evidence of the terrible condition of things became apparent. The first thing in the shape of a vehicle that I saw was a truck, loaded with coffins, going around to collect the dead. As this was within four blocks of the depot you may imagine how soon I came to a realizing sense of the desolation. Two blocks further on, coffins were piled in tiers on the sidewalk in front of the undertaker's shop, and we were compelled to walk between them. . . . Everyone was thoroughly frightened, a young doctor said to me. "It takes a man of great moral courage to stay in this place. You talk with a man tonight and tomorrow hear that he is in the grave."

The summer of 1878 was hot and wet. Accordingly, the 1878 attack of yellow fever was so virulent that those physicians who had witnessed the epidemic five years earlier thought they were confronted by a new, deadlier strain of yellow fever. In this assessment they were likely correct. Even the African Americans, usually resistant to yellow fever, also succumbed as never before, with over 11,000 infected, or 77 percent of their population in Memphis. Their illness was generally more severe than in previous epidemics, and their mortality was considerably higher at 10 percent, although much lower than the 70 percent death rate among Caucasians (of the 6000 that remained, more than 4000 died).

Many victims of this plague died alone covered with the black vomit characteristic of the disease. Whole families were wiped out. For example, Mrs. Barbara Flack, a widow, and all her seven children, from twenty-eight to three years of age, were killed. A nun helping in the care of the sick noted:

> Carts with 8 to 9 corpses in rough boxes are ordinary sights. I saw a nurse stop one day and ask for a certain man's residence. . . . The Negro driver just pointed over his shoulder with his whip at the heap of coffins behind him and answered, "I've got him here in this coffin" (17).

The Surgeon General, Dr. John M. Woodworth of the U.S. Marine Hospital, reported, "Scenes enacted here during the height of the epidemic would seem more appropriate to the domain of sensational fiction then to the serious pages of a medical journal; but the facts come under my own observation."

Doctors had enormous loads of patients and were mentally and physically exhausted. One wrote, "I wish I could go to some secret spot where there would be no burning heads and hands to feel, nor pulses to count, for the next six weeks. It is fever, fever all day long and I am weary. . . . . I do not know what to think or do. . . . Nothing but distress and death on all sides" (19).

In an attempt to understand the cause of this disease and how to treat it, physicians performed about 300 autopsies. But afterward, they knew little more than they had before: "We can write and talk learnedly of epidemics and other forms of disease but when in the midst of a visitation . . . we are so overwhelmed with our impotence, and the unsatisfactory result of treatment" (20).

Yellow fever did not seem to be directly transmitted by person-to-person contact or by food or drinking water. Although germs were the suspected cause, attempts to demonstrate the agent had failed. Was yellow fever spread by inhalation of infected air? What were the conditions, so far unidentified, that allowed the disease to spread? What were the local sites where this disease occurred, and why was there an association with a warm climate. These questions had no answers in 1878.

The Memphis telegraph office kept lines open to other parts of the nation. Informed of the plight, states in the North, South, East, and West quickly sent supplies and funds. Then yellow fever struck those in the telegraph office as well. Of the thirty-three men in the Memphis office, nineteen died.

With the frosts of October 18 and 19, and a concomitant decrease in the mosquito population, the rate of yellow fever infection dropped rapidly. The epidemic was declared over on October 29. Refugees came home to seek the graves of lost friends and relatives. On Thanksgiving day, the city of Memphis held a mass meeting to praise the heroes of the epidemic, to thank the rest of the nation for its help in sending assistance, and to mourn the dead. There were fewer than 20,000 who remained in the city, and of these over 17,000 had gotten yellow fever. Of the 14,000 African-Americans, roughly 11,000 got the fever and 946 died. Of the 6,000 Caucasians, nearly all got yellow fever and 4,204 died. Although the epidemic of 1878 hit Memphis most severely, throughout the Mississippi Valley over 100,000 had the fever and 20,000 died (20).

In the fight to control and prevent yellow fever, several groups of microbe hunters stand out. The first group, represented by Dr. John Erskine, serves as a model of those health care workers who gave their lives caring for infected patients. There were 111 known physicians in Memphis, of which seventy-two came from other states in the country. All were fully aware of the risks

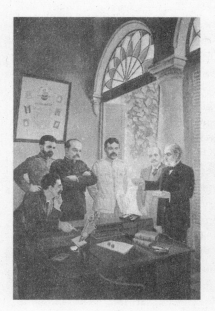

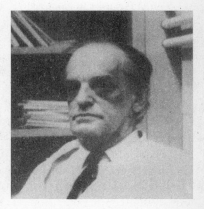

Figure 5.3 The conquerors of yellow fever. (Left) *A painting of Carlos Finlay with the members of the Yellow Fever Commission, Walter Reed, James Carroll, Jesse Lazear (all in uniform), and Aristides Agramonte (not shown). Both Carroll and Lazear were to become infected by yellow fever, with Lazear dying from the disease.* (Right) *Max Theiler, who developed the 17D yellow fever strain vaccine that conquered the epidemic form of the disease.*

involved, but they were determined to stay. Most had not had yellow fever before and so had no immunity to the disease. More than 60 percent gave their lives caring for patients during this epidemic. The second group was comprised of Jesse Lazear, James Carroll, Aristides Agramonte, and Walter Reed of the United States Army Yellow Fever Commission, who were appointed in 1900 and led by Reed. Within this group, Lazear, Carroll, and Agramonte risked their lives by self-experimentation, documenting that yellow fever was a transmissible agent passed by the *Aedes aegypti* mosquito from patient to patient. The third group was characterized by Max Theiler, who successfully attenuated the yellow fever virus and developed a strain (17D) that allowed vaccination and prevention of the disease.

John Erskine was born in Huntsville, Alabama, in 1834 and became a Memphis Health Officer. At the height of the plague, when the city was one of silence and death, Erskine's fearlessness, his abundant energy, and his tireless work to treat victims were noted by his contemporaries. During those weeks when only doctors, nurses, relief workers, undertakers, and grave diggers were active, he was considered a model of the best medical professionals. A graduate of New York University Medical School in 1858 and a Confederate surgeon during the American Civil War, he returned to Memphis in 1865 and played an active role in the yellow fever epidemics of 1867, '73, and '78. He was chosen Health Officer of the city in 1873, '76, and '78. It was in his capacity as Health Officer in 1878, while treating sufferers of yellow fever, that he became infected and died. In spite of the raging plague, fifty leading citizens united and provided a tribute to his memory (13,18). Simultaneously, local and national newspapers eulogized him and his work. In 1974 the city of Memphis named one of its libraries for him and filled its shelves with accounts of the city's health disasters and triumphs. In 1990, St. Jude's Hospital in Memphis established an annual lectureship in his honor.

Twenty years after the death of John Erskine, during the last years of the nineteenth century, Reed, Lazear, Carroll, and Agramonte, under the auspices of the United States Yellow Fever Commission, performed experiments on human volunteers in Havana to identify the source of yellow fever (21–25). Their results demonstrated clearly that the blood of patients with yellow fever was infectious during the first three days of fever, that *Aedes aegypti* mosquitos feeding on the patients during those three days became capable of transmitting the infection after an interval of about twelve days, and that the infectious agent in human serum passed through a Berkefeld filter, indicating it was a virus, not a bacterium. These experiments also proved that yellow fever was not transmitted by fomites (inanimate objects or materials capable of conveying disease-producing agents), and that disinfection of clothes and bedding was unnecessary, because this disease was not passed by patient-to-patient contact. From this work, Walter Reed and his coworkers are credited with establishing that the agent of yellow fever is a virus. Mosquitos ingest the viruses when they bite and draw blood from an infected human and then, after a lag period, expel these viruses into the blood of new victims by biting them.

Walter Reed was born in 1851 in rural Belroi, Virginia, where his father was a Methodist minister. At the age of seventeen, he became the youngest graduate of the University of Virginia Medical School. He continued his medical education at the Bellevue Medical School (now New York University Medical School) from which he received his medical degree. After several years of work in various New York hospitals he joined the United States Army and was commissioned, in 1875, as an Assistant Surgeon. After the next fifteen years spent at various Army posts, he took a sabbatical leave and went to the newly established Johns Hopkins Medical School in Baltimore. During this time, he became acquainted with William Osler, considered the most illustrious physician in North America, and trained in pathology and bacteriology with William Welsh. Welsh had earlier studied in the newly emerging bacteriology laboratories in Europe established in response to the observations of Koch and Pasteur. In 1893, Reed was made curator of the Army Medical Museum and appointed Professor of Bacteriology at the recently established Army Medical School.

In stark contrast to Reed, James Carroll was a freespirit who described himself as a "wandering good-for-nothing." He was born in England, and left at age fifteen for Canada. There he lived as a backwoodsman until enlisting in the United States Army. He decided to become a physician while serving as a hospital orderly at Fort Custer, Montana. With encouragement from Reed, he studied initially at Bellevue Medical College in New York and received his medical degree from the University of Maryland School of Medicine in Baltimore. He then also trained in bacteriology and pathology at the Johns Hopkins Hospital with William Welsh. In 1897, Carroll became Reed's laboratory assistant. In this same year, at the urging of George Sternberg, then Surgeon General of the Army Medical Corps, Reed formed and headed a Commission to do research on yellow fever, and Carroll became second in command.

The two civilian physicians, Jesse Lazear and Aristides Agramonte, attended Columbia University Medical School in New York but came from very different backgrounds. Jesse Lazear was born in 1866 to a wealthy family in Baltimore. Trained in art as well as medicine, he also traveled to Europe where he studied modern bacteriologic techniques. After receiving his medical degree in 1892, he became the first Chief of Clinical Laboratories at the Johns Hopkins Medical School and joined the Yellow Fever Commission in that position. He was described as "quiet, retiring and modest." The other civilian physician was Aristides Agramonte. He was born in Cuba and brought to New York City as an infant after his father was killed in an abortive revolt to free Cuba from Spain. Described as "energetic and nosy," he worked as a bacteriologist for the New York City Health Department after obtaining his medical degree. He joined the Yellow Fever Commission as a civilian pathologist in charge of laboratories at Military Hospital #1 in Havana and was Chief Physician on the yellow fever ward.

Yellow fever was endemic in Cuba and thus endangered all countries with whom Cuba traded. In 1898, with the outbreak of the Spanish–American War, yellow fever became a primary concern of the United States Army. Therefore, the Yellow Fever Commission was sent to Cuba in 1900. Interestingly, at that time, none of the four members had observed a case of yellow fever previously. Their first aim was to confirm or refute the claim that yellow fever was caused by a bacterium, namely *Bacillus icteroides*, as first proposed by Guiseppe Sanarelli, an Italian pathologist who injected the bacteria into five South American subjects of whom three died from jaundice. Although the conclusion that bacteria caused yellow fever brought Sanarelli notoriety and awards, the Yellow Fever Commission proved the idea untrue. The bacillus had simply been a contaminant, a passenger in patients with yellow fever; it was not the cause. The Commission then turned their investigation to the hypothesis of Carlos Finlay (26–28) that a mosquito was the transmitter of yellow fever.

Carlos Finlay, born in Camaguey, Cuba, was the son of Scottish and French parents. He entered the Jefferson Medical College in Philadelphia in 1853, a year in which yellow fever caused considerable disease in that city. This episode, in addition to the multiple cases occurring in Cuba, focused his interest and laid the foundation for his life's work in the investigation of yellow fever. He graduated from Jefferson Medical College in 1855, and in 1857 began the practice of medicine in Havana. In 1881 Finlay formally presented his thesis, "The Mosquito Hypothetically Considered as the Agent of Yellow Fever" (26). In this report he concluded that, since yellow fever affected vascular endothelium, a blood-sucking insect might be an intermediate host responsible for transmission. He described three events necessary for the transmission of yellow fever:

1) The existence of a yellow fever patient into whose capillaries the mosquito was able to drive its stinger and impregnate it with virulent particles,

at an appropriate stage of the disease. 2) That the life(cycle) of the mosquito be spared after it bites a yellow fever patient and so it has a chance of biting the patient in whom the disease is to be reproduced. 3) The coincidence that some of the persons whom the same mosquito happens to bite thereafter shall be susceptible of contracting the disease.

Consistent with other discoveries throughout the course of medicine and science, the concept that a mosquito causes yellow fever had earlier been suggested by many but proven by none. For example, in 1807 John Crawford of Baltimore published a paper stating that the mosquito was responsible for malaria, yellow fever, and other diseases, and in 1848 Joshua Nott from Mobile, Alabama, reiterated this concept. An interesting side-line is that Dr. Nott, in his function as an obstetrician, delivered William Gorgas, who in the 1900s would virtually eliminate the *Aedes aegypti* mosquito from Cuba and other areas throughout the Americas including the site where the Panama Canal was to be built. In 1853 Louis Beauperthuy, a French physician working in Venezuela, also incriminated the mosquito in spreading yellow fever and malaria. However, none of these physicians provided any experimental evidence to confirm the hypothesis. To the contrary, Finlay undertook realistic experimentation. First, he trapped wild mosquitoes and allowed them to bite yellow fever patients and then bite healthy individuals who had no previous history of yellow fever. However, the results were inconclusive. Although four of the five healthy individuals became feverish and mildly ill, classic yellow fever did not occur. Indeed, the Army Surgeon General, William Sternberg, one of the premiere microbiologists in North America and the organizer of the Yellow Fever Commission, totally rejected Finlay's experiments and the mosquito theory. Having worked directly with Finlay in Cuba during the first Yellow Fever Commission of the late 1870s, Sternberg respected the work of Finlay but believed that mosquitoes did not inject anything harmful into humans. Unfortunately, Sternberg's position of power was sufficient to dampen support for Finlay's hypothesis. Nevertheless, evidence was mounting that insects could indeed transmit disease to man (28). In 1878, Patrick Manson found that a mosquito infected humans with the parasitic disease filariasis. Theobald Smith in 1892, along with Frederick Kilbourne, showed that ticks spread the parasitic disease of cattle called "Texas Fever." In 1894, Manson showed that the tsetse fly caused human sleeping sickness or trypanosomiasis, and in 1896, Ronald Ross of the British Army showed that mosquitoes transmitted malaria.

The Yellow Fever Commission members differed in their opinions as to whether the mosquito could cause yellow fever, with Lazear being the only one among the four who strongly believed so. No animal except man was known at that time to be susceptible to yellow fever. Therefore to test the mosquito transmission hypothesis, members of the commission decided to engage in human experimentation. None were enthusiastic about taking the risk of catching yellow fever, but Carroll, Lazear, and Agramonte directly participated. Reed did not. To control these studies, they reared the mosquitoes from eggs provided by Carlos Finlay so as to rule out the mosquitoes' previous exposure to humans or to any human disease. In the first set of experiments, Lazear and eight other volunteers were bitten by mosquitoes almost immediately after they had bitten patients with yellow fever. As described by Agramonte:

> Each insect was contained in a glass tube covered by a wad of cotton, the same as is done with bacterial cultures. As the mouth of the culture is turned downwards, the insect usually flies towards the bottom of the tube (upwards), then the bottom is uncovered rapidly and the open mouth placed upon the forearm or abdomen of the patient; after a few minutes the mosquito drops upon the skin and if hungry will immediately start operations; when full, by gently shaking the tube the insect is made to fly upward again and the cotton plug replaced without difficulty.

None of the nine individuals came down with yellow fever.

Next, Carroll volunteered for experimentation: "I reminded Dr. Lazear that I was ready, and he at last applied to my arm an insect that had bitten a patient with a severe attack 12 days previously. . . . I was perfectly willing to take a soldier's chance." That night Carroll wrote Reed, who had returned to Washington, "I remarked jokingly, that if there were anything in the mosquito theory I should have a good dose, and so it happened."

Two days later Carroll experienced the earliest vague symptoms of yellow fever and four days later the symptoms became severe, marked by weakness, chills, and a temperature of $102°F$. No malaria parasites were found in the blood that came from Carroll, ruling out the possibility of malaria. Agramonte wrote:

> Not finding any malaria parasites, he (Carroll) told me he thought he had caught a cold at the beach; his suffused state, bloodshot eyes and general appearance in spite of his efforts at gaiety and unconcern, shocked me beyond words. Having yellow fever did not occur to him. Lazear and I were almost panic stricken when we realized that Carroll had yellow fever.

Carroll's life was in the balance. He was delirious with fever fluctuating between 103°F and 104°F, severe headache, back pain, swollen gums, yellowing of his eyes and body. However, he did not bleed severely and within several days his temperature was normal.

The relief in Carroll's survival from yellow fever is dramatically recorded in the letter sent to him from Walter Reed, who was in Washington at the time of Lazear's and Carroll's illness:

Sept. 7, 1900
1:15 pm

My Dear Carroll:
Hip! Hip! Hurrah! God be praised for the news from Cuba today—"Carroll much improved—Prognosis very good!" I shall simply go out and get boiling drunk!
Really I can never recall such a sense of relief in all my life, as the news of your recovery give me! Further, too, would you believe it? The Typhoid Report is on its way to the Upper Office! Well, I'm damned if I don't get drunk twice!
God bless you, my boy.

Affectionately,
Reed

Come home as soon as you can and see your wife and babies.
Did the mosquito do it?

Carroll's attack left him so weak that two weeks later he could not stand or change position without assistance. However, Carroll had been in contact with yellow fever patients a few days immediately preceding his illness, so it was not clear whether the mosquito bite alone had caused the yellow fever or had been an incidental factor. For that reason, the next experiment was done on a volunteer who had no previous exposure to yellow fever, Private William H. Dean. On the day that Carroll became sick, Lazear applied to Dean's arm, in addition to three other mosquitoes, the same mosquito that had bitten Carroll, to provide the greatest chance of transmitting the disease. But Dean developed only a mild case of yellow fever. So, on September 13, 1890, Lazear let himself be bitten again. Five days later he began to feel ill. As the disease progressed, Lazear developed jaundice, vomited blood, and became delirious. Just 12 days after the experiment began, Jesse Lazear died.

James Carroll wrote, "I shall never forget the expression of his eyes when I last saw him alive on the third or fourth day of his illness."

Washington D.C.
September 26, 1900

My Dear Carroll:

Major Kean's cable, telling of poor Lazear's desperate condition, was quickly followed by the one announcing his death—I cannot begin to express my sorrow over this unhappy termination of our colleague's work!

I know that your own distress is just as acute as my own—He was a brave fellow and his loss is one that we can with difficulty fill. I got the General to cable yesterday about securing Lazear's notes which he wrote that he had taken in each case bitten by mosquitoes.—Examine them carefully and keep all.

I will leave here in the morning for New York—and will ask you to meet me with a conveyance at the foot of O'Reilly Street or at the Navy yard dock if you can find out from Quartermaster where passengers will land on the arrival of the Crook, which should be Wednesday, October 3.

If your observations are such as you and Lazear have intimated, we must publish a preliminary note as soon as it can be gotten ready.

Affectionately,
Reed

The evidence was now substantial. Yellow fever was transmitted by mosquitos, and a lag time was required between the insect's acquisition of infected blood and biting of a susceptible individual to induce disease. This latter point accounted for the failure of Finlay's experiments and of Agramonte's first attempt to become infected. This time lag after the mosquito first feeds on the blood of a subject with the yellow fever virus is twelve to twenty days, during which the virus travels from the insect's gut to its salivary gland, a position where the virus is available to infect the next susceptible individual. This timing agrees with that observed by Henry Carter, a U.S. Public Health Service physician who in 1898 conducted epidemiologic studies of yellow fever in two Mississippi villages. He concluded that an extrinsic incubation period of approximately two weeks was required for the induction of new cases of yellow fever.

Thus, of the four Commission members who undertook the study of yellow fever in Cuba, one died and another barely survived. Their conclusion that the mosquito served as an intermediate host for the agent of yellow fever and that disease was propagated through the bite of this insect was not universally accepted, however. For example, the *Washington Post* on November 2, 1900, in publishing the mosquito hypothesis reported, "Of all the silly and

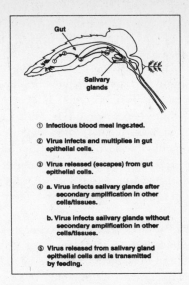

Gut

Salivary
glands

① Infectious blood meal ingested.

② Virus infects and multiplies in gut
epithelial cells.

③ Virus released (escapes) from gut
epithelial cells.

④ a. Virus infects salivary glands after
secondary amplification in other
cells/tissues.

b. Virus infects salivary glands without
secondary amplification in other
cells/tissues.

⑤ Virus released from salivary gland
epithelial cells and is transmitted
by feeding.

Figure 5.4 The life cycle of the yellow fever virus in the
mosquito. Schematic courtesy of Fields' Virology *(Philadelphia:*
Lippincott-Raven, 1996).

nonsensical rigmarole of yellow fever that has yet found its way into print—
and there has been enough of it to build a fleet—the silliest beyond compare
is to be found in the arguments and theories generated by a mosquito hypothesis."

Shortly thereafter, on November 20, the Yellow Fever Commission members established another experimental camp in Cuba. Strict quarantine was
enforced and experiments conducted only on subjects never previously
exposed to yellow fever. Named Camp Lazear, the facility was created to
include only residents who were judged to be susceptible to yellow fever and
with no previous exposure to the disease. Of five volunteers tested, four contracted the disease, but all recovered. The one volunteer who did not get sick
was bitten by a mosquito later found incapable of transmitting the infection.
The irrefutable conclusion was: "The precision with which the infection of
the individuals followed the bite of the mosquito left nothing to be desired."

To fulfill the exacting requirements of scientific experimentation, additional research was performed and clearly showed that yellow fever was not
spread by human-to-human contact, or spread through fomites and was transmitted by the injection of blood taken from infected patients into susceptible

humans. Further, when the infectious blood was passed through a filter designed to retain bacteria, it still transmitted disease, indicating it was not bacterial in origin.

One consequence of these studies was that William Gorgas, Chief Sanitary Officer in Havana, introduced anti-mosquito measures that decreased the number of yellow fever cases in Havana from 1400 in the year 1900 to none in 1902. The second consequence was the building of the Panama Canal. Results from the United States Yellow Fever Commission deserve much of the credit for preventing this disease in the large labor force needed to build a ship route across the tropical isthmus of Panama, joining the Atlantic and Pacific Oceans. The third and lasting consequence was that the days of ignorance, superstition, and controversy about yellow fever and its transmission were over.

The building of the Panama Canal was first conceived and undertaken by Ferdinand de Lesseps, born in 1805 into a family of wealth and national service (29,30). His interest in canal building is believed to have begun in Egypt in 1830. An interesting figure, his drive to build two great ship canals through the isthmus of Suez and the isthmus of Panama were attributed more to his almost religious drive to achieve great events for France and the welfare of humanity than to any prospect of financial gain.

To undertake the challenge of building the Panama Canal (29–32), the Compagnie Universelle du Canal Interoceanique raised funds for the "La Grande Entreprise," the biggest financial venture ever attempted at the time. French engineers of the nineteenth century were an exceptional breed and took the task of building the canal as a matter of French pride and destiny. At the beginning of 1881, some 200 French or European engineers and some 800 laborers began making test moorings on the isthmus, also building barracks, hospitals, and roads. They actually began chopping a pathway across Panama. Lacking knowledge of the cause of yellow fever and the breeding habits of mosquitoes, they used large pots with stagnant water in gardens and under the legs of barracks and hospital beds, to retard trafficking by ants. These water vessels provided an exceptionally good milieu for the breeding of mosquitos. By the end of 1881 over 2000 men were at work and the digging of the great trench began. In 1882, approximately 400 deaths were reported, and in the next year 1300 from yellow fever and malaria. Approximately 200 laborers died each month. Reports of the death rate in Panama were so frightening that they were suppressed to assure financial stability in France and to continue raising funds by bond issues for building the canal. However, reports began filtering back to France as sons who participated in the Panama challenge died there. Engineering schools soon began advising their graduates against going to Panama. Nevertheless, graduating engineers continued to answer the call for this grand adventure in Panama, "as officers hastened to the battlefield and not as cowards who flee from the sorrows of life." However, the project became more difficult and hazardous as unexpected earthquakes and landslides added to the deaths from yellow fever. For example in 1885, of seventeen newly graduated French engineers arriving in Panama, only one survived the first month.

To stem the rumors of death from yellow fever, Jules Dingler, in charge of the Panama Canal operation, brought his entire family to Panama. This move was designed to provide the best possible proof of the Director General's confidence in Panama. But within several months, his only daughter contracted yellow fever and died within a few days. His wife wrote to Charles de Lesseps:

> My poor husband is in despair which is painful to see—my first desire was to flee as far as possible and carry far from this murderous country those who are left to me. But my husband is a man of duty and tries to make me understand that his honor is the trust you have placed in him that he cannot fail in his task without failing himself. Our dear daughter was our pride and joy.

A month later Dingler's remaining child, a son of twenty-one, showed signs of yellow fever and in three days he too was dead. Dingler wrote to de Lesseps:

> I cannot thank you enough for your kind and affectionate letter. Mme. Dingler who knows that she is for me the only source of affection in this world, controls herself with courage, but she is deeply shaken. . . . We attach ourselves to life in making the canal our only occupation; I say "we" because Mme. Dingler accompanies me in all my excursions and follows with interest the progress of the work.

Shortly thereafter their daughter's fiancé died in Panama, also of yellow fever, and by summer forty-eight officers of the canal company were also dead. In Paris the fearful death toll was no longer secret. Engineers, physicians, nuns, and laborers sent to work on the canal were developing yellow fever. Patients were dying so swiftly and so desperate was the need for bed space that in the final minutes of life, a dying man saw his own coffin brought in. For the sick who never made it to the hospital—the vast majority—the end was frequently more gruesome:

> Sitting on your veranda late in the evening you see the door of a little adobe house across the way open. The woman of the house, who lodges

two or three canal employees, peers cautiously out in the street, reenters the
house, and when she comes out again drags something over the threshold,
across the narrow sidewalk, and leaves it lying in the dirty street. When she
closes the door again there is no noise but the splash of the tide.... Soon it
grows lighter. A buzzard drops lazily down from the roof of the cathedral
and perches on something in the street. The outlines become more distinct.
You walk down, drive away the bird who flies suddenly back to his watch-
tower, and stand looking in the quick dawn of the tropics at what was yesterday a man—a month before a hopeful man, sailing out of Le Havre. He
is dead of yellow fever.

So wrote a visitor from the *Herald Tribune*, S. W. Plume. He would recall, "It
was the same way—bury, bury, bury, running two, three, or four trains a day
with dead all the time. I never saw anything like it. It did not matter any difference whether they were black or white, to see the way they died there."
The rate of sickness was not determined accurately, but a conservative estimate was that about one-third of the total work force at any given time was
infected with yellow fever. Thus in a year such as 1884, with more than
19,000 at work, probably 7,000 were sick.

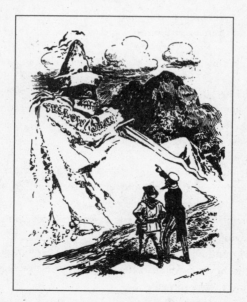

*Figure 5.5 A cartoon from the early 1900s indicating a principal
challenge to Theodore Roosevelt and the United States government on
building the Panama Canal.*

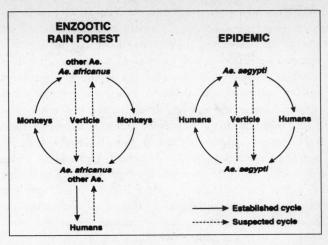

Figure 5.6 The spread of yellow fever: various host-mosquito life cycles. Modified from Fields' Virology *(Philadelphia: Lippincott-Raven, 1996).*

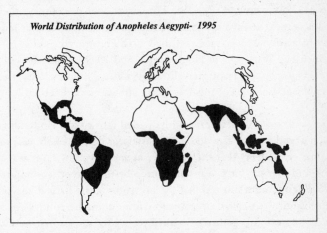

Figure 5.7 The theoretical danger of spread of yellow fever today is depicted on this world map that displays (in black) the current habitat of the mosquito vector of yellow fever. Illustration courtesy of Brian Mahy, Centers for Disease Control, Atlanta, Georgia.

By December 1888, the news of continued sickness and death associated with yellow fever, coupled with rising costs, led to a financial crash. Publicity about these overwhelming risks prevented the company formed to dig the canal from raising new capital, and it dissolved by February 1889. Within a few years, the United States government, led by Theodore Roosevelt, reinstated the challenge to connect the Atlantic and Pacific Oceans (3,32,33). By this time the Yellow Fever Commission report was known, and the success of William Gorgas in controlling both yellow fever and malaria in Havana through mosquito eradication well established. By overcoming the disease, medical scientists paved the way to success for this engineering project.

Although the *Aedes aegypti* mosquito clearly transmitted yellow fever throughout the Americas, researchers soon learned that other mosquitoes could transfer disease in jungle populations (3,4). Further, experimentation showed that monkeys could be infected and were susceptible hosts of yellow fever, so instead of being conquered and eliminated, this disease continues to pose a considerable and permanent threat. With rapid air travel and other transportation, the possibility of bringing yellow fever into urbanized areas remains real, especially since the *Aedes aegypti* mosquito still lurks on the borders of the southern United States and is prevalent throughout Mexico and the Caribbean. Thus, in still another way, the story of yellow fever is not yet complete.

A third and more recent group of microbe hunters were those at the Rockefeller Foundation (3,34–38). For over half a century, they have mounted a comprehensive and broad attack on yellow fever that led to the discovery of a yellow fever vaccine called 17D. This group, guided by Wilbur Sawyer, included Wray Lloyd, Hugh Smith, and Max Theiler. It was Theiler who built on the discovery of the yellow fever virus, attenuated its effects, and developed a safe vaccine. For this innovation, he was awarded the Nobel Prize in 1951 (39).

The research on yellow fever can be divided into two periods. During the first, Walter Reed and his coworkers in Havana, as described above, proved by using human volunteers that the causative agent of yellow fever was a filterable virus, and that the virus was transmitted by the bite of a common urban mosquito. Then Gorgas showed that by interrupting the habitat and breeding of these mosquitos, so-called urban yellow fever could be controlled.

The second period began nearly thirty years after the U.S. Army Commission's work in Havana when, in 1928, Adrian Stokes, Johannes Bauer, and N. Paul Hudson (34) of the Rockefeller Foundation found that rhesus monkeys were susceptible to yellow fever virus, thus providing the first animal model of this disease. Later the first strains of the yellow fever virus family were isolated—the Asibi and the French Dakar strains. Despite the accumulated knowledge about yellow fever, this disease continued to kill, including those microbe hunters working with the viruses. Stokes, Hideyo Noguchi, and William Young, members of the Commission, subsequently died from yellow fever.

Eventually scientists realized that, although urban yellow fever could be controlled by elimination of the *Aedes aegypti* mosquito, they could not exterminate the so-called jungle yellow fever carried by mosquitoes in the canopies of tropical trees along with the virus's natural host, the monkey. Unfortunately, this life cycle of yellow fever viruses in mosquitos and monkeys could be and was occasionally interrupted when man entered the habitat, contracted yellow fever, and brought it to the outside world. This remains so today.

In the laboratory, Max Theiler developed a small animal model of yellow fever infection that was easier to work with than the rhesus monkeys formerly used. He was able to show that intracerebral inoculation of Swiss white mice with the yellow fever virus caused disease. This discovery simplified study of the disease and eventually its control. Mice could be protected from a lethal injection of yellow fever if they first received sera from humans or monkeys that were immune to the disease. Theiler then established a method of testing for antibodies to the virus in the blood stream, charted the epidemiology of the disease, and finally provided the framework for attenuating or disarming the virus, a necessary requirement for the development of a successful vaccine.

Beginning in 1927, when yellow fever virus was isolated from a patient named Asibi in the African Gold Coast, scientists recorded the movements of this virus in monkeys and intermittently in *Aedes aegypti* mosquitos. Later they tracked its passages in embryonic cultures. At some point in the culture passages the virus mutated and lost its ability to produce fatal encephalitis, a disease of the central nervous system, when injected into rhesus monkeys and later even into mice. Eventually this virus caused monkeys to make antibodies within five days. These antibodies protected them so that later injection with the virulent Asibi strain of the yellow fever virus did not cause the disease. The next step was the vaccination of laboratory personnel working with yellow fever. Afterward, although the vaccinees experienced mild side-effects, they made antibodies that neutralized the virus—the basis of immunization. The end result was production of the 17D strain of yellow fever virus (37–39). Thereafter, over 59,000 people were vaccinated with 17D and 95 percent of these showed immunity against yellow fever. Subsequently, millions have been vaccinated with successful results. Recently molecular biology techniques used to identify the amino acid sequences of this virulent Asibi and the 17D vaccine strains located differences in only thirty-two amino acids of the two strains. Exactly what has mutated in the virus to cause its attenuation is not known but may be in a protein of its outer layer.

Max Theiler's background positioned him uniquely to work with the yellow fever virus. He was born in January 1899, one year after the formation of the U.S. Army Commission on Yellow Fever. As a child in Pretoria, South

Africa, under the influence of his family, he became an observer of the animals and plants around him. He received his medical training at the University of Basle and Cape Town but completed his studies at St. Thomas' Hospital in London. Thereafter he took a short course in tropical medicine and hygiene at the London School of Tropical Medicine. This experience focused him on an area of biomedical research that held his interest for the rest of his scientific career. While still in London, he met Dr. O. Teague of Harvard Medical School, who recruited Theiler to join a group there under the direction of Andrew Sellards at the Harvard Medical School. In 1930, Wilbur Sawyer induced Theiler to leave Harvard and join the Rockefeller Foundation in New York, where in 1937 he developed the 17D strain of yellow fever vaccine. In 1951 he was awarded the Nobel Prize for "discoveries concerning yellow fever and how to combat it."

Despite the effectiveness of the vaccine, yellow fever still lurks in any area frequented by *Aedes aegypti* mosquito. With the introduction of just one person infected with yellow fever, the disease could once again emerge as a terrifying plague. Further, yellow fever is unlikely to be completely exterminated like smallpox has been and measles and poliomyelitis may be, because the virus remains part of a monkey-mosquito life cycle in the world's jungles. Rapid travel to and from those jungles makes it possible that yellow fever may emerge once again. Since World War II, outbreaks of yellow fever have been documented in Western Panama, with a spread through Central America to the southern borders of Mexico. Elsewhere, yellow fever afflicted Trinidad, Ethiopia, Senegal, Nigeria, and the upper Volta region in Sierra Leone, Ghana, and elsewhere. The 1960–62 outbreak in Ethiopia alone involved an estimated 100,000 persons and caused 30,000 deaths in a population of one million. Although mass vaccination reaching at least 90 percent of a population should be able to control outbreaks, yellow fever remains endemic in countries adjacent to the equatorial forests of the Amazon basin in South America. The *Haemagogus* mosquito, which also transmits yellow fever, lives in this jungle region, and the *Aedes aegypti* mosquito still dwells throughout parts of south-central Latin America, Mexico, and along the southwest and southeast border of the United States. Yet now that we have a more perfect understanding of the disease, its route of transmission, and methods to control epidemics, the unrelenting fear of yellow fever that was present 100 years ago is no longer with us. Still, to grasp the hysteria of that time, one needs only to focus on the disease Ebola, which currently arises periodically in Africa. Ebola (see Chapter 10) is a "new" viral hemorrhagic fever with a high rate of fatalities, but little is known about its natural history, how it is transmitted, whether it has non-human hosts, when it will appear, or how it can be stopped.

CHAPTER 6

MEASLES VIRUS

When measles virus attacks people who for generations have been isolated from exposure to the virus, nearly everyone becomes infected and many die. By this means whole native tribes have been nearly obliterated. An example is Fiji, which was placed under administrative rule by the British Colonial government in the last half of the nineteenth century. To participate in signing the Colonial Treaty, the Chief of the Fiji people, Thacombau, traveled to Sydney, Australia. During the voyage home aboard His Majesty's ship Dido, on January 6, 1875, one of Thacombau's sons and a native attendant became ill and developed measles. Treatment followed the isolation procedures of the time, so the two patients were kept separate from the crew by quarantine in a temporary house built on the ship. By January 12, when the boat arrived at the native city of Levuki, both patients recovered and went ashore. But on January 14 and 15, another of Thacombau's sons came down with measles. Yet with festive plans already in place, on January 24 and 25, the other native chiefs, their retainers and their relatives from all the nearby islands met in a great assemblage to learn of the treaty and to pay their respects to Thacombau. After two days of celebration they returned to their separate villages. Just thirteen days later, on February 12, an epidemic of measles erupted. By February 25, the British authorities enforced quarantine regulations throughout the islands. However, all the Chiefs and subjects throughout their villages were now ill. According to William Squire (1), a physician in the area, "All the Chiefs who attended the meeting have it and it is spreading rapidly."

By March 13, "The attacks have been so sudden and complete that every soul in the village is down with it at once, and no one able to procure food or if procured cook it for themselves or others. . . . People have died of starvation and exhaustion in the midst of plenty." In the ensuing four months there were more than 20,000 deaths from measles, and the native population was depleted by over 40 percent.

Seventy-seven years later, with the availability of precise laboratory tests to complement clinical observations that documented the presence of measles, an epidemic was recorded in southern Greenland (2). The attack rate of measles virus in this virgin population was 99.9 percent, with a mortality corresponding to that seen earlier in the Fiji islands. The vaccine to conquer measles was still eleven years in the future, and the only treatment available then as in the past was supportive therapy, providing nourishment and food in a quiet environment.

Measles virus is transmitted through the air (3,4). Infected droplets are released by talking, coughing, and sneezing. These measles viruses sprayed into the air reach cells lining the mouth, throat, nose, and eyes of potential victims. The lower respiratory tract (lungs and bronchi) are more susceptible to infection than the nose-to-throat canal, which is in turn more susceptible than the mucous lining of the mouth. During the initial two to four days after infection, the virus replicates in local areas of the respiratory cells and spreads to draining lymph nodes where a second round of viral production occurs. The virus then enters the bloodstream carried within white cells of the blood (leukocytes and peripheral mononuclear cells). The end result is viruses circulating in the blood (viremia) and carrying infection to many parts of the body. The infected person feels well; during this time there is little obvious clinical evidence of viral infection, although the viruses permeate the body. Thus, the initial measles virus infection and incubation periods are silent.

The next (prodromal) phase of measles begins after the eight to twelve day incubation period and is heralded by fever, weakness, and loss of appetite. This is followed within a few hours by coughing and running of the eyes and nose. Along with this phase is a second interval of viremia, greater in magnitude

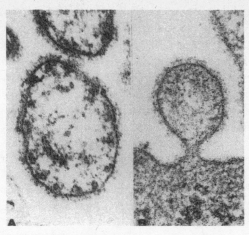

Figure 6.1 Electron micrographs of measles virus particles (virions). Magnification, 120,000x. (Left) *The complete virion composed of an envelope covered by a fuzzy outer coat (virus glycoproteins) and lined on the inside by fuzzy nucleocapsids. The nucleocapsid contains the viral RNA. When cut in cross-sections the measles virus matrix protein, located under the plasma membrane, has a donut appearance.* (Right) *A virion budding from the plasma membrane of an infected cell. Studies and photomicrographs by Michael B. A. Oldstone and Peter W. Lampert.*

than the first, that spreads infection to tissues throughout the body. These viruses are again carried primarily within mononuclear cells, and it is the further replication of virus in these cells together with development of the host's specific attack against the viruses (immune response) that are responsible for the signs and symptoms of disease. These signs and symptoms reflect involvement of cells lining the respiratory tract, the gastrointestinal tract, and the eyes. In addition, as cells in small blood vessels become infected and interact with components of the host's immune response (antibodies and T cells), the characteristic measles virus rash begins on the face and spreads rapidly over the body, arms, and legs.

The cough increases in intensity as does the fever, reaching its peak on about the prodromal fifth day. The rash begins after the third or fourth day and consists of small 3- to 4-mm red maculopapular (flat to slightly raised) lesions that blanch on pressure. Characteristically the rash appears first behind the ears and on the forehead at the hairline, then spreads downward over the face, neck, upper extremities, and trunk, and continues downward until it reaches the feet by about the third day after its first appearance. Soon it begins to disappear.

However, the immune system is often crippled during this phase (3–5). The intense inflammation of lymphoid tissues and cells that comprise the immune system suppresses the ordinarily vigorous immune function required to control other non-measles infections. Other microbial diseases normally held in check by a functioning immune system are now able to rage in some patients. It is this virus-induced suppression of the immune system, first recognized in the late 1800s, that is responsible for many of the deaths during measles virus epidemics, although measles viruses by themselves, as a consequence of inducing infection, are also capable of causing death.

Measles virus was the first infectious agent known to abort the immune response, leaving humans susceptible to other microbial agents. This ominous picture is all too familiar today as redefined by the human immunodeficiency virus (HIV), and the acquired immunodeficiency syndrome (AIDS) epidemic that HIV continues to cause (5).

Once measles virus infection was accurately identified, several interesting consequences followed. During the nineteenth century, tuberculosis was rampant. Observers of the disease recognized that infected persons could progress to the terminal stage and die, or enter a stage of arrested illness only to have full-blown tuberculosis recur at a later time. In the absence of anti-tuberculosis drugs, which were not developed until around the mid-twentieth century, the preferred therapy was simply rest, in the countryside or in a sanitarium located in a quiet place, preferably at high altitude. Near the end of the nineteenth century, clinicians attending these patients recognized that, following a measles virus infection, arrested tuberculosis became active and spread rapidly through the body (6). Patients with syphilis reacted similarly; measles caused reactivation and rapid spread of the formerly arrested disease.

The Austrian pediatrician Clements von Pirquet developed a cutaneous, or skin, test for tuberculosis and he noted that (7): "A positive reaction to the tuberculin test signifies that the individual has been in contact with tubercular bacillus. . . . It is not possible, however, to conclude directly from that finding in which stage of tuberculosis that the individual is; the disease may be either active and progressive or inactive." However, this reaction to tuberculosis can be transiently lost, as von Pirquet noted: "the cutaneous reaction in tuberculosis that had been present can disappear following measles virus infection" (7). Von Pirquet recognized that measles virus infection suppressed the host's immune response, as noted by loss of the immune response to tuberculin. This loss of immunity allowed the reemergence of clinically active tuberculosis. At the beginning of the twentieth century, many medical practitioners knew that virus infection could suppress the immune system and that a secondary or other microbial infection, either newly involved in infecting the host or one

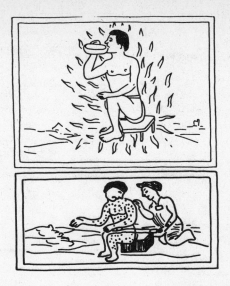

Figure 6.2 Measles virus victim in this sixteenth-century Aztec drawing from the Códue Florentino.

that was maintained in an inactive stage, would then become rampant. Another interesting observation of von Pirquet's was that patients with active kidney disease (nephrosis) who would ordinarily die from kidney failure were protected and the clinical disease temporarily halted after they became infected with measles virus (8). Although why this occurred was not fully understood, similar and multiple observations with measles virus and nephrosis led some physicians to treat nephrosis by purposely infecting the patients with measles virus (9). In fact, in patients with autoimmune kidney disease, the immune system was aggressive against the body's own tissues, and by suppressing the immune response by use of measles virus, the process of nephrosis was halted. With the invention of cortical steroid hormones to suppress the immune system, this viral therapy was discontinued.

Suppression of the immune system induced by measles virus infection, especially in undernourished and genetically susceptible individuals, left the patients open to continuing reinfection by any of several passing bacteria. Affected sites were primarily the lungs, producing pneumonia, and the intestinal tract, causing diarrhea, both of which contributed to a high death rate. Such events decimated the Indian tribes of North, Central, and South America (10,11). A graphic example is the deaths of Aztecs and Peruvian

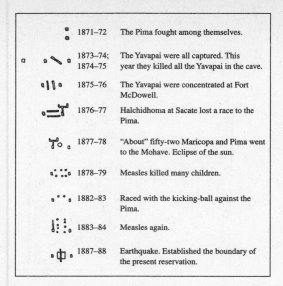

	1871–72	The Pima fought among themselves.
	1873–74; 1874–75	The Yavapai were all captured. This year they killed all the Yavapai in the cave.
	1875–76	The Yavapai were concentrated at Fort McDowell.
	1876–77	Halchidhoma at Sacate lost a race to the Pima.
	1877–78	"About" fifty-two Maricopa and Pima went to the Mohave. Eclipse of the sun.
	1878–79	Measles killed many children.
	1882–83	Raced with the kicking-ball against the Pima.
	1883–84	Measles again.
	1887–88	Earthquake. Established the boundary of the present reservation.

*Figure 6.3 Sticks/stone messages of different dates from the Yuma tribes
of the Gila River and the role measles virus infection played in their lives.
From Leslie Spie,* Yuma Tribes of the Gila River *(New York:
Cooper Square, 1970).*

natives during the Spanish conquest of South and Central America; measles
killed these populations along with smallpox, as described in Chapter 4.
Another example is the Yuma tribes of the Gila River in southern Arizona.
This community of native Americans indicated significant occurrences in
their lives by marking sticks with scratches and dots between dash marks that
denoted the year of an event of importance (12). Selected elderly people of
the tribe made these records. By such artifacts their history has been traced
from 1838, with references to measles in 1878–79 and 1883–84 (12).
Although other illnesses undoubtedly struck them over this timespan, only
measles is recorded, presumably because of its devastation among the tribes.

There is no treatment that arrests measles virus infection, once begun. To
control its spread to others in a susceptible population, until the 1960s, quarantine (13) or the segregation of infected persons was the only protection
known. Until the vaccine to control measles arrived in 1963, measles continued to wreak havoc on peoples throughout the world. For example, during the
pre-vaccine era in the United States, each year there were approximately four
million cases with 48,000 of them requiring hospitalization and 500 dying. A
serious complication was infection of the brain, or encephalitis, in 4,000 per-

sons, of whom 1,000 had permanent brain damage and deafness. In some instances the viruses led to a chronic, progressive neurologic disease in which loss of brain function eventually ends in death, usually within seven to ten years following infection (3). Currently, the estimated annual cost from injury and death by measles virus infection in the United States was $670 million (4).

Normally, recovery from measles virus infection produces a lifelong protection from reinfection (14). This conclusion was reached by a young Danish medical officer, Peter Panum, when studying the outbreak of measles virus in the Faeroe Islands in 1846 (15). In March 1846, a carpenter to be employed in the Faeroes left Copenhagen, Denmark, shortly after visiting friends ill with measles. He arrived eight days later in the village of Thorohavn. On April 1 he developed measles. Before the end of that year, 6,000 cases were documented amongst the 7,782 inhabitants. Because the Faeroes were under Danish control, Peter Panum, in his capacity as a Medical Health Officer, was dispatched from Denmark to assist in the fight against this epidemic. He noted that the measles virus infected only individuals younger than sixty-five years of age (15). The high attack rate in all others from early infancy to sixty-five years matched closely the data from a previous outbreak of measles in 1781. Thus, he reasoned, persons who were resistant to the current Faeroes epidemic of 1846 had been exposed to measles virus sixty-five years earlier. Panum based his firm conclusion on three facts. First, the Faeroe Islands were isolated. Second, quarantine of all ships prior to their docking and allowing crews to come ashore was strictly enforced. Third, the number of ships landing in the Faeroes over that sixty-five year span was limited. Panum was able to accurately define the incubation period between the last and current attacks of measles virus, the infectiousness of the illness in newly afflicted individuals, and the duration of immunity among individuals who had earlier contracted measles virus. This observation of lifelong immunity after infection, coupled with the fact that humans were the only host for measles virus infection—that is, no animals carried the virus—would be an important guide and stimulus to John Enders and his colleagues who 100 years later created the measles vaccine. This vaccine, by preventing the disease, eventually provided the means for eliminating measles.

When introduced into isolated, relatively small communities, measles virus attacked with disastrous consequences. Further, the infection of rural populations not previously exposed to childhood illnesses led to untold consequences especially during war times and with the forced migration of peoples. The American Civil War was the last large-scale military conflict fought before the germ theory of disease was developed by Louis Pasteur, Robert Koch, and Joseph Lister. Two-thirds of soldiers who died in that war, 660,000 in all, were killed by uncontrolled infectious diseases. Of these, in the Union Army over 67,000 had measles and more than 4,000 died.

In the early years of the Civil War, the strategy of Abraham Lincoln and his war cabinet focused upon the rapid seizure of Richmond, Virginia, led by George McClellan in the Peninsula Campaign. However, disease attacked McClellan's army along the Chickahominy River, reducing his troop strength by over one-third. Several hard-fought battles against the Confederate Army of northern Virginia led for the first time by Robert E. Lee stalemated the Union Army's efforts, forcing McClellan to abandon the project and retreat (16–18). During this first year of war there were 21,676 reported cases of measles and 551 deaths in the Union Army alone. Deaths were primarily from respiratory and cerebral (brain) involvement. It was recorded, "This affection is always serious, often fatal either directly or through its sequelae. The prognosis therefore should be guarded"(18).

Measles also ravaged the Confederates with over 4500 sick at Winchester, less than three weeks after the battle of Antietam. Lee wrote to the Secretary of War:

> They are principally, if not altogether, the conscripts and recruits that have joined since we have been stationary. They are afflicted with measles, camp fever, etc. The medical director thinks that all the conscripts we have received are thus afflicted, so that, instead of being an advantage to us, they are an element of weakness, a burden. I think, therefore, that it would be better that the conscripts be assembled in camps of instruction, so that they may pass through these inevitable diseases, and become a little inured to camp life.

And to his wife:

> We have a great deal of sickness among the soldiers, and now those on the sick-list would form an army. The measles is still among them, though I hope is dying out. But it is a disease which though light in childhood is severe in manhood, and prepares the system for other attacks. The constant rains, with no shelter but tents, have aggravated it. All these drawbacks, with impassable roads, have paralyzed our efforts (19).

At this time America was primarily a rural society. Newly formed regiments with many susceptible soldiers from the countryside had their first exposure to the contagious diseases of childhood in the camps of assembly. Measles virus was the chief offender. Because of the solid immunity following an attack, most knowledgeable commanders "seasoned" their troops before sending them as reinforcements for battle. "Well-seasoned troops" were soldiers who had survived the epidemics that struck most recent enlistees. Typical was the response of General M. Lovell to a request from Richmond that he forward new troops from New Orleans in January 1862 (16). He would send them, "as soon as [he] can have them put through the measles; a process which they are now undergoing—one-half of them now being sick" (20).

It was the congregation of sufficient numbers of susceptible individuals that promoted measles virus outbreaks in the Civil War. Measles virus was and is primarily a disease of large cities. Urbanization brings in close contact large groups of people which are a requirement for maintaining the measles virus pool. Aggregations of people permit the continuous circulation of viruses and provides a balance between an abundance of the virus and a continuous supply of susceptible individuals. Epidemiologic studies suggest that a population of 200,000 is required to sustain measles virus infection (21, 22). With increasing urbanization, measles virus shifted away from an illness of adults to primarily a disease of children—now the most susceptible targets of infection.

It is likely that the great river valley cultures, dominant over 6000 years ago in Mesopotamia and along the Tigris–Euphrates Valley, were the first to suffer measles virus epidemics. Indeed, it has been debated that the plague of Athens in 4 B.C., in Antonine of the Roman world in the second century A.D., in China in 162 and 310, and in Tours in southern France in the sixth century were associated with or consequences of measles virus infection (10). The formation of these urbanized centers as large, complex, organized, and densely populated cities brought together diverse people, some with resistance and others with susceptibility to measles virus.

How measles first came to infect humans is not clear. Perhaps the source was animal herds brought together in close proximity with large groups of people. The similarities between measles virus and canine distemper virus (3) of dogs and rinderpest virus (3) of cattle make the latter viruses suspects in the development of measles virus infection. This concept has long been fancied but never proven. Definitive proof is hard to come by, as the identification of measles virus infection was difficult to distinguish from smallpox virus infection. Consequently both had been lumped together as a single entity. It was in the tenth century that the Arab physician Abu Becr (also called Rhazes) first attempted to distinguish between smallpox and measles (23). But not until the seventeenth century did the English physician Thomas Syndenham (24) actually document the clinical entity of measles infection. From that time forward accurate records of the disease and its effect on populations accumulated. The movement of large populations to cities, attracted by job opportunities of the industrial revolution, ensured the continuous presence of measles virus and cycling of the disease. The disease was identified as a virus in 1911 (25), when respiratory secretions of a patient with measles virus were passed through a filter designed to retard bacteria but allow the passage of viruses. Inoculation of the passaged fluids into monkeys then caused a measles-like disease. Many observations have indicated that the natural host for measles virus is man, and among the animal species only certain primates are susceptible to this infection. Interestingly, monkeys are not infected by measles virus in their natural habitat. They become infected only when they come in contact with humans incubating the virus. Perhaps the small tribal social structure of monkeys allows this susceptible population to avoid measles virus infection in nature.

Once it was understood that infection with measles virus confers lifelong protection from the disease and that man is the natural host, interest turned toward developing a preventative vaccine. The principles of growing bacteria in culture had been defined in the mid- and late-nineteenth century by Robert Koch and Louis Pasteur. Such cultivation techniques allowed the isolation of the causative bacterial agents in pure cultures. This allowed investigators to manipulate, purify, and do biochemical and biological studies on bacteria. For example, the ability to grow bacteria in the culture dish and in the test tube was instrumental in the discovery of antibiotics, which have reduced bacterial infections dramatically. In addition, therapeutic materials such as inactivated toxins, antibodies to toxins, and vaccines were produced in this way. Thus, devastation by the bubonic plague, cholera, typhoid, diphtheria, sepsis, endocarditis, and meningitis was largely prevented by the products of laboratory research. Such products reduced deaths from bacterial infection by over 99 percent.

The situation was different for viruses. Viral diseases, except for smallpox and yellow fever, mentioned earlier, remained largely unabated. Viruses, unlike bacteria and other microorganisms, replicate only inside living cells. Therefore, the inability to grow viruses in culture became the main limitation to controlling such viral infections as measles and poliomyelitis. In the first decade of the twentieth century, Alex Carrel had developed a procedure for growing cells in culture. Interestingly, Carrel worked with Charles Lindbergh, the aviator who was the first to fly across the Atlantic Ocean, on the development of the artificial heart and was awarded the Nobel Prize in 1912 for his work on "vascular suture and the transplantation of blood vessels and organs." However, it was Carrel's pioneering work with tissue culture (27) that was to be of more interest. Unfortunately, his methodology was burdensome, difficult, and impractical. Then in the 1920s S. Parker, Jr., and R. Nye showed that viruses could grow and multiply in cultured tissue. It was Hugh and Mary Maitland who simplified this technique and kept cell fragments alive in culture for short periods of time (28).

Hugh Maitland was born in Canada and, after training in bacteriology at the University of Toronto and in Germany, worked at the Lister Institute on the first animal virus isolated, foot-and-mouth virus. In 1927 he was appointed to the Chair of Bacteriology at the University of Manchester, England. There, with Mary Cowan Maitland, he succeeded in growing vaccinia virus in a simple tissue culture system, later known as Maitlands' medium. This suspended cell technique of the Maitlands was applied extensively by multiple investigators to the study of viral growth.

Thus in 1936, Albert Sabin and Peter Olitsky attempted to grow poliomyelitis viruses in Maitland cultures of tissues from chick, mouse, monkey, and human embryos. However, they found that only in the human embryonic brain tissue would the virus replicate. Their conclusion, that the virus was strongly neurotropic (attracted to nerve cells) and that growing of poliovirus was not practical or possible in other cell types, as we will see in Chapter 7, was incorrect, but was reasonable at the time. For their studies, Sabin and Olitsky used a poliovirus obtained from Simon Flexner of the Rockefeller Institute that was likely already adopted and restricted for growth in nerve cells. This virus had multiple passages through the monkey nervous system. The reversal of this misconception was accomplished by Thomas Weller, Frederick Robbins, and John Enders, who used human embryo cultures in the isolation of varicella virus (a DNA virus that causes chickenpox) and viruses from cases of diarrhea. They used a different source of poliovirus to infect these cells (29, 30). John Enders was destined to develop the measles virus vaccine.

John Franklin Enders was born in 1897 to a family of means in West Hartford, Connecticut. Beginning in a graduate program of English at Harvard, he focused on English and Celtic literature. However, impressed by the teaching of Hans Zinsser, Chairman of Bacteriology and Immunology at the Harvard Medical School, he decided to pursue a Ph.D. course in microbiology. Three years later, at age thirty-three, he received his doctorate degree in bacteriology and immunology and was appointed an instructor at Harvard Medical School. Like most microbiologists of his generation, he worked on tuberculosis and pneumococci, studying how to control infection by these microbes. A devastating disease of kittens that rampaged through the animal quarters at Harvard in 1937 grabbed Enders's attention and changed the direction of his future field of study. Enders, with William Hayman, showed that the cats had a

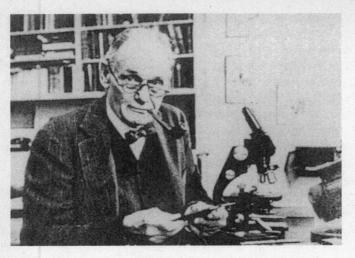

Figure 6.4 John Enders, whose group at Harvard developed the effective attenuated live measles virus vaccine.

disease caused by a filterable agent and that this agent could transmit the disease. These observations on what proved to be panleukemia virus of cats provided Enders with his first real experience in virology, led to his first publication in this field, and focused the remainder of his career on this discipline. It was also at this time that Enders, working with the tissue culture techniques of the Maitlands, realized their unsuitability and returned to Alex Carrel's approaches for growing cells in tubes that slowly rolled (roller tubes). In spite of this method's complexity, he was successful by the 1940s in growing large amounts of vaccinia virus in cultured cells and obtaining high titers of virus. He was also able to prolong the lives of grown chick embryo cells in culture. This work was interrupted by the Second World War, after which Enders returned to Harvard where a research division of infectious disease was established at the Children's Hospital for his continued work. The major theme of his endeavors was to be the application of tissue culture techniques to virology and the extension of his findings to diagnosis and prevention. With his newly improved techniques, he repeated the Sabin–Olitsky studies in 1946 but used tissue-culture cells. He showed that poliomyelitis viruses grew in brain tissue, but also in cultured cells from the skin, muscles, and intestines. He then proved that viruses produced in this way caused recognizable cytopathology (cell destruction) and that serum from the blood of individuals who were immune to poliovirus could block such cell destruction. Now Enders was able to supply virologists with a tool as important as the one Pasteur and

Koch had provided for bacteriologists by developing defined culture media. Viruses could be grown in culture, isolated, purified, and attenuated.

Fifty years before Edward Jenner (31) showed that cowpox inoculation protected humans against smallpox and introduced the concept of vaccination, and thirty years after Lady Mary Montagu had her son variolated in Constantinople (32), a Scottish physician, Francis Home (33), had had the same idea and attempted to produce mild measles by mimicking the variolation process. This process involved taking blood from an infected patient and inoculating it through the skin of an uninfected person. In this way he was able to transfer measles to ten of twelve patients. This experiment clearly demonstrated the presence of measles virus in human blood nearly 100 years before Frosch and Loeffler described the first animal virus (32). With the availability of a roller tube culture system and knowing of Home's results, Enders and his student Thomas Peebles obtained viruses from the blood and throat washings of a youngster, David Edmonston, who had an acute measles virus infection, and grew these viruses in epithelial cells obtained from kidneys of humans and monkeys (35). These viruses, subsequently grown in human kidneys, human amnionic fluid, fertile hen eggs, and chick embryo cell cultures, became the progenitors for the vaccines used today. For recognizing and adapting the culture method for replicating viruses, mainly poliomyelitis virus, Enders, with his colleagues Frederick Robbins and Thomas Weller, received the Nobel Prize in 1954.

The safety of cultured and attenuated viruses in producing immunity but not disease was demonstrated first in monkeys. Viruses passed in cultured cells were selected for their diminished ability to harm recipients while still inducing an immune response upon inoculation. Monkeys injected with the tissue culture–passed live viruses soon developed protective antibodies. When these viruses were inoculated into monkeys intracerebrally (into the brain), no disease or tissue damage occurred. By contrast, monkeys not first immunized developed severe measles virus infection when exposed to the virus. After this success, the attenuated virus was tested in humans, first by inoculating the vaccine into immune adults in whom it was safe. The next step was a bigger clinical trial using children in several American cities. The results were dramatic. In 1961 Enders and his colleagues reported that measles virus infection could be prevented through vaccination (4).

Shortly thereafter, in September 1961, the *New York Times* wrote an editorial enthusiastically complimenting Enders on his accomplishment in developing the vaccine for measles and his work leading to the development of the poliomyelitis vaccine (36). Enders's response, published on October 1, 1961 (37), epitomizes what is the best in and of science:

To the Editor of the *New York Times*:

Editorial reference was made to our work on measles and poliomyelitis in your edition of Sept. 17. I wish to express my deep appreciation of these favorable comments on our work.

For the sake of accuracy, however, I would emphasize the fact that whatever may have been accomplished represents the joint product of many co-workers supported by several institutions. In the studies on measles virus and vaccine, essential contributions were made by Thomas C. Peebles, Milan V. Milovanovic, Samuel L. Katz, and Ann Holloway. In the researches on the growth of polio virus the role of Thomas H. Weller and Frederick C. Robbins was as important or more important than my own.

Without the generous provision of financial aid and physical facilities not only by Harvard University but also by the Children's Hospital Medical Center, Boston, the National Foundation, the Armed Forces Epidemiological Board, the United States Public Health Service and the Children's Cancer Research Foundation, in which a large part of our laboratory is situated, nothing could have been done.

To me it seems most desirable that the collaborative character of these investigations should be understood, not solely for personal reasons but because much of all modern medical research is conducted in this way.

John F. Enders
Professor of Bacteriology and Immunology at the Children's Hospital
Harvard Medical School
Boston, Sept. 20, 1961

The widespread vaccination of children in the United States and other countries has had a dramatic effect on the incidence of measles virus and its complications. A single exposure to the measles virus vaccine results in the production of antimeasles virus antibodies in 95 to 97 percent of susceptible individuals. However, an unsolved problem remaining has been those infants infected with measles virus before their ninth month of age (4). This early infection occurs in a number of countries where the virus continues to circulate widely, particularly in the sub-Saharan African nations. The nine-month period is a window of susceptibility between the time those children lose protection afforded by passage of the mother's antibody through the placenta to the fetus and the time when attenuated viruses in the vaccine successfully replicate. The mother's antibody obtained by breast feeding, although protective to the newborn, inactivates the attenuated virus vaccine. Whether this dilemma will be overcome by immunization of all susceptible children and adults, thereby reducing the circulating virus pool, or design of a new vaccine

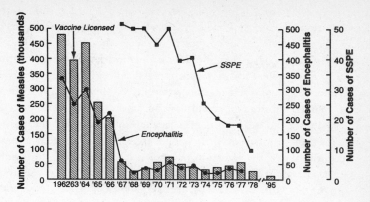

Figure 6.5 The effect of measles virus vaccine in controlling cases of acute measles virus infections (hatched bars). Acute brain (encephalitis) and chronic brain (subacute sclerosing panencephalitis, a chronic progressive degeneration of the brain) complications are shown.

that can provide protection and not be neutralized by maternal antibody, remains to be determined. This conflict is currently being hotly debated among experts on measles virus infection (in favor of providing an additional vaccine that would not be neutralized by the mother's antibody) and epidemiologists (mainly in favor of using the current vaccine only). The outcome will have an important impact on the goal of eradicating the measles virus.

In addition to the large numbers of infants under a year of age who are susceptible to infection, a considerable population of children and adults lack immunity to the measles virus. The virus circulates in a community until its chain of transmission is broken by massive vaccination. Unless this occurs within a short period of time, control is not likely to be achieved. However, as documented for the treatment of measles in Gambia from 1967 through 1970, measles can be brought under control. In this instance, before the onset of mass vaccinations, there were 1,248 documented cases, but in 1969 and 1970 that number was reduced to zero following a series of universal vaccinations done each year. What is clear from such examples is that a commitment by all nations to enforce a program of immunization with the current vaccine will reduce the presence of circulating virus in most areas of the world.

Another problem still remaining is the significant number of vaccine recipients who fail to respond to the initial vaccine dose. To counteract this difficulty, many countries have instituted a two-dose schedule, with a second dose given at varying times after the first one. With such a strategy, measles has been eliminated entirely in Finland, Sweden, and Cuba, and the annual number of reported cases in the United States reduced from more than two million per year to less than a few hundred. However, the virus is highly contagious and still travels beyond the borders from countries where vaccination is universal to those where it is not widely practiced, and measles viruses continue to infect those who remain susceptible. Other countries have made vaccination voluntary instead of mandatory. In Japan, despite some difficulties experienced with the side effects of a Japanese-manufactured measles virus vaccine, the vast majority of their people have been vaccinated and, until recently, outbreaks of the infection numbered less than a few thousand per year. However, within three years of abolishing the mandatory requirement for taking measles virus vaccinations, over 200,000 cases of measles developed in Japan during 1995–1997.

In Third World countries, the elimination of measles is more difficult to achieve than in developed countries because of the higher contact rates and reproduction rates as well as the less well-developed infrastructure to provide vaccination. But even in highly industrialized countries like the United States, measles has not been eliminated. The cause is the inadequate vaccination coverage in preschool-age children and the approximately 5 percent primary vaccine failure rate.

The World Health Organization (WHO) estimates that in the 1980s and early 1990s as many as 2.5 million children died annually from measles, primarily because of the failure to vaccinate susceptible individuals. With prodding from WHO and other health organizations, 78 percent global coverage by measles immunization was achieved, so that reported cases dropped significantly and deaths were reduced by over 70 percent to an annual rate of approximately one million.

The WHO in 1990 set the goal of "reduction by 95% in measles deaths and reduction by 90% of measles cases compared to pre-immunization levels by 1995 as a major step towards the global eradication of measles." Eradication is planned by the second decade of the twenty-first century. Since humans are the only reservoir for measles virus, immunity provides lifelong protection, and immunity can be induced by vaccination, WHO is justified in proposing global eradication of measles virus. Measles, once the scourge of all lands, is now controlled in most, although it still currently kills millions in developing countries. The strategy for elimination of this virus depends on the dedication of every government to cleansing the world of this infectious agent.

With rapid travel to all parts of the world, those coming from areas where measles virus still circulates provide a hazard to susceptible people in distant countries. Measles viruses infect approximately 40 million children and kill more than one million of them a year worldwide. The will to save these one million-plus lives per year and the finances required rest solely on the dedication, responsibility, and commitment of the more fortunate nations on this planet and, in turn, on the politicians and legislatures responsible for setting priorities. Whether measles-related deaths will continue for over 100 years after the development of the measles virus vaccine, as was true for the smallpox vaccine, will largely be determined by the kind of society present in the twenty-first century.

CHAPTER 7

POLIOMYELITIS

On April 12, 1955, church bells pealed throughout the United States. Employees of the National Foundation for Infantile Paralysis beamed, and thousands upon thousands of volunteers for the lay organization the March of Dimes celebrated a job well done. These volunteers had walked their communities, apartment houses, cinema theaters, and even grocery stores soliciting contributions, and millions of adults and school children had made large and small donations. Not since the Second World War had the fabric of America been woven together more tightly in a single cause. That cause was the conquest of poliomyelitis. The ringing of the bells was testimony to the announcement that the clinical trial of the polio vaccine showed it to be effective in preventing disease. The Associated Press dispatch of that day read: "(Advance) Ann Arbor, Mich. (AP)—"The Salk polio vaccine is safe, effective and potent it was officially announced today."

Diseases, in general, have no respect for the boundaries of any one nation or region. However, with polio, two countries made it their own challenge.

Epidemics in the late nineteenth and early twentieth century in Scandinavia, where outstanding clinical investigations and epidemiologic studies by Karl Oskar Medin, Ivor Wickman, Karl Kling, and others took place, led to a lasting commitment by Sweden toward the understanding and treatment of polio. The second country to make such a stand was America. A major epidemic in New York City and surrounding cities during 1916 riveted attention on this disease. Five years later, the man who was to be the thirty-second President of the United States, Franklin Delano Roosevelt, became paralyzed from the waist down after infection with the poliomyelitis virus in mid-life. Formation of the National Foundation for Infantile Paralysis, primarily by Basil O'Connor and other friends of Roosevelt, coupled with the mounting concern of parents that their children would become victims of this crippling disease and the belief that infantile paralysis might be conquered, led to an American crusade to fight polio. With missionary zeal throughout all parts of the United States, dimes and dollars were raised to alleviate the suffering and tragedy polio inflicted and to wipe out the infectious virus that was responsible. It was one of the rare times, outside of war, in which the citizenry of a nation was united. The result was one of medicine's greatest technical and humanistic triumphs, indicating what is possible when public support, science, and technology are directed to the good of humankind. This commitment to eliminate poliomyelitis virus from the world by the year 2000 continues today through the World Health Organization and support of the Rotary International.

Unlike other viral diseases that began waning or remained constant in the twentieth century, poliomyelitis was on the increase. In the United States it blighted lives with increasing epidemics that peaked in 1952, during which time nearly 58,000 became sick, 21,000 were paralyzed, and over 3,000 died. In 1954, just one year before the pealing of the bells, more than 38,000 individuals were infected (1,2). The impact of poliomyelitis was felt not only in the United States but worldwide. Epidemics were common in Asia, South America, Europe, and elsewhere. In fact, in the early 1950s it was the fifth major killer of young children in Sweden (3). For as long as any parent or child could remember, each summer brought fear that a poliomyelitis epidemic would sweep through and indiscriminately kill the young and healthy or cripple survivors, leaving them a legacy of withered limbs and destroyed ambitions. Not until the National Foundation for Infantile Paralysis proved successful in its quest for a vaccine to prevent poliomyelitis did country-wide vaccination cause the number of cases to drop below 1,000 in 1962, below 100 in 1972, and to fewer than five by 1992. The natural virus has not caused a single case of poliomyelitis in the United States during the last decade; the few cases (5 to 10) recorded per year are the result of a side effect of using a live vaccine.

The stories of poliomyelitis and of three main personalities who were fundamental in development of the vaccine for its conquest, Jonas Salk, Albert Sabin, and Hilary Koprowski, are the subjects of this chapter. Jonas Salk and his colleagues chemically inactivated the poliomyelitis virus with formaldehyde and provided a vaccine that produced immunity and dramatically lowered the incidence of poliomyelitis (2, 4). Salk became the people's hero in the war on polio. But immunity, in terms of antibody quantities produced by the inactivated vaccine, waned over time. Additionally, administration by needle made vaccinations of large populations difficult. For these and other reasons, Koprowski, Sabin, and others independently worked on the development of vaccines with live attenuated (weakened) viruses, following the successful examples of Jenner's smallpox vaccine and Theiler's yellow fever vaccine. The attenuated vaccines developed by Sabin and Koprowski also proved highly effective in large clinical trials on humans (2, 5–7). The Sabin vaccine was chosen over the Koprowski vaccine and in most countries replaced the Salk vaccine. Sabin never enjoyed the popular glory that Salk received but obtained the scientific respect that Salk never got. Koprowski's achievements in the development of the polio vaccine, for the most part, were forgotten. Yet all three played important roles in the victory over the plague of poliomyelitis. There were many others, of course, who made seminal contributions. Without such efforts the vaccine would never have been developed. To mention but a few, best known are work on the monkey model by David Bodian, Isabel Morgan, and colleagues, epidemiologic and clinical studies by John Paul, Dorothy Horstmann, and William Hammon, tissue culture studies by John Enders, Thomas Weller, and Frederick Robbins, and the immunologic observations of Macfarlane Burnet.

Paralytic poliomyelitis epidemics first became known in the nineteenth century. Whether or not sporadic outbreaks of paralytic poliomyelitis occurred earlier is less certain and a matter of disagreement (2,6). The de-scription of Ramses's withered limb as a child in ancient hieroglyphic records is inadequate to associate the deformity with an infection, but poliomyelitis virus is a possible cause. Similarly, the priest pictured with a withered leg on an Egyptian stele of the fifteenth to thirteenth century B.C. is characteristic and reminiscent of a deformity caused by poliomyelitis infection but, of course, could have originated from trauma, birth defect, vascular insufficiency, or other afflictions. Numerous other examples of withered limbs were known in antiquity and throughout the Middle Ages (2,6). However, polio, which could have been responsible, was not defined as a specific disease entity until the late seven-

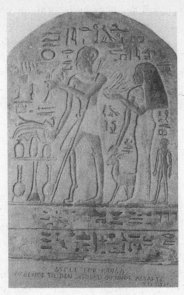

Figure 7.1 The earliest known illustration of a suspected case of poliomyelitis. An Egyptian stele dating from the eighteenth dynasty (1580–1350 B.C.).

teenth century. It was at that time and through efforts of Thomas Sydenham (8), an English physician who lived from 1624 to 1689, that symptoms described by patients and signs documented by their doctors were correlated and classified with specific diseases. On occasion such correlations came only at autopsy. This early devotion to charting clinical details was the basis for sorting fevers, rashes, and so on, into defined clinical entities and diseases. Hence, if poliomyelitis did occur before 1800, its incidence was sporadic and not in the epidemic forms of the nineteenth century.

The late eighteenth century and early nineteenth century provides us with good examples of what was probably paralytic poliomyelitis. The great Scottish writer and poet Sir Walter Scott, who was born in Edinburgh in 1771, developed an attack of fever in infancy that left him permanently lame, as in the following description of his own illness:

I showed every sign of health and strength until I was about 18 months old. One night, I had been often told, I showed great reluctance to be caught and be put to bed, and after being chased about the room, was apprehended and consigned to my dormitory with some difficulty. It was the last time I was to show much personal agility. In the morning I was discovered to be effected with the fever which often accompanies the cutting of large teeth. It held me three days. On the fourth, when they went to bathe me as usual, they discovered I had lost the power of my right leg. My grandfather, an excellent anatomist as well as physician, the late Alexander Wood, and many others of the most respectable of the faculty, were consulted. There appeared to be no dislocation or sprain; blisters and other topical remedies were applied in vain.

When the efforts of regular physicians had been exhausted, without the slightest success, my anxious parents, during the course of many years, eagerly grasped at every prospect of cure which was held out by the promise of empirics, or of ancient ladies or gentlemen who considered themselves entitled to recommend various remedies, some of which were of a nature sufficiently singular.

The impatience of a child soon inclined me to struggle with my infirmity, and I began by degrees to stand, to walk, and to run. Although the limb effected was much shrunken and contracted, my general health, which was of more importance, was much strengthened by being frequently in the open air, and, in a word, I who was in a city and probably being condemned to helplessness and hopeless decrepitude, was now a healthy, high-spirited, and, my lameness apart, a sturdy child.

The lameness, coming on suddenly and unexpectedly in a child, after a short bout of fever, makes this a suspected case of poliomyelitis. Similar cases may have also been frequent at this time, but most often doctors were not called early enough and, when called, were consulted only after the child had been lame for weeks or months.

It was left to Michael Underwood (9) in 1789 to provide one of the earliest known, accurate descriptions of the clinical picture of paralytic poliomyelitis: "debility of the lower extremities, usually attacks children previously reduced by fever . . . when both [limbs] have been paralytic, nothing has seemed to do any good but irons to the legs, for the support of the limbs, and enabling the patient to walk."

Underwood refers not to any epidemic but only to isolated cases. Later, in 1840, the German physician Jacob Heine (10) wrote the first review that described several patients with the disease and its clinical characterization. By 1870, Jean-Martin Charcot (11) applied microscopic study to tissues obtained from patients with poliomyelitis, noting the shrinking and loss of substance in the anterior horn of the gray matter of the spinal cord—the area containing the large motor neurons that control the limbs.

Charles Bell was a Scottish physician whose unique feats of observation were well appreciated by many, including Arthur Conan Doyle, who modeled, in part, his detective Sherlock Holmes after him. Bell wrote what is probably the first description of an epidemic of poliomyelitis depicting events in 1844 on the island of St. Helena (12):

A lady whose husband was the English clergyman at St. Helena consulted me about her child, who had one leg much wasted. In conversing about the illness, which preceded this affliction in her little girl, she mentioned that an epidemic fever spread among all the children in the island about three or five years of age; her child was ill of the same fever. It was afterwards discovered that all the children who had the fever, were similarly affected with a wont of growth in some parts of their bodies or limbs! This deserves to be inquired into.

From the time of Bell's recorded observation, reports of epidemics of poliomyelitis were confirmed and on the increase. Numerous Swedish investigators contributed significantly toward the characterization of poliomyelitis. Oskar Medin characterized poliomyelitis as an acute infection, and Ivor Wickman, his student, published several studies of poliomyelitis epidemics.

The modern push to solve the poliomyelitis problem described by Medin and Wickman had its origins during the last third of the nineteenth century. Revolutionary concepts formed by Louis Pasteur and Robert Koch, their students, and a host of eager disciples established the foundation of bacteriology, immunology, and virology. These scientists dispelled the then current doctrine of "spontaneous generation," which held that all kinds of lower forms of life arose de novo in some mysterious way from materials in which they were usually found, for example, maggots from rotting flesh. The revolution resulted in the discovery and isolation of infectious agents and the assignment of their roles as the sources of specific diseases. These early bacteriologists made culture media in which to grow isolated bacteria and used the microscope to identify the microbes that grew in the media. Through a porcelain-type filter connected to a hand pump, fluids obtained from such cultures or samples obtained from patients, animals, or plants were passed to collect bacteria. These first filters, known as Pasteur-Chamberland-Berkefeld-type filters, contained several standard pore sizes, the smallest of which excluded bacteria from passing through. The bacteria collected on such a filter could be grown in culture, studied, and analyzed. However, in contrast, certain infectious materials did pass through the filters. Although these materials were invisible under the microscopes of the time and would not grow in culture media, they did multiply when reinoculated into appropriate laboratory or domestic animals. This was the first method of isolating viruses.

The infectious agent that causes foot-and-mouth disease in cattle was the first virus to be isolated from an animal. Friedrich Loeffler and Paul Frosch passed fluid obtained from vesicles of cows with an unknown disease into the Pasteur-Chamberland filter. Whereas bacteria were retarded by the filter, the infectious agent causing foot-and-mouth disease passed through (13). This material would not grow in culture medium. However, when inoculated into infection-free cows, it reproduced foot-and-mouth disease. Four years earlier Dmitri Ivanoski's observed a filterable agent obtained from the tobacco plant and known as tobacco mosaic virus. From the turn of the twentieth century until the outbreak of World War I, filtration devices were actively applied to the isolation of viruses.

The events of Karl Landsteiner's career in the laboratory moved polio research toward its successful conclusion. After graduating from the Medical School at the University of Vienna in 1891, Landsteiner spent five years studying chemistry in several laboratories outside of Austria, including that of the great German chemist Emil Fischer in Wurzburg. Landsteiner returned to Vienna to assume a junior faculty position, the same year that Loeffler and Frosch discovered foot-and-mouth virus. In 1908, during an epidemic of poliomyelitis in the city of Vienna, Landsteiner, along with Edwin Popper, obtained spinal cord material from a nine-year-old boy who had died of the disease. Landsteiner then tried to infect a series of animals with this material. At that time, the cause of poliomyelitis, whether from an infection or not, and, if so, by what agent, bacteria or virus, was unknown. Inoculations of rabbits, guinea pigs, and mice did not result in any illness. But fortune smiled on these two experimentalists. They wanted to test their material on monkeys because of their physiologic similarity to humans, but then, as now, monkeys were expensive and available only in limited numbers. Two Old World monkeys were offered to Landsteiner and Popper for transmission studies because the monkeys were so-called "damaged goods," since they had been used previously for other experiments. These monkeys were deemed expendable. In contrast, unused New World monkeys were on hand but reserved for higher ranking professors and more important projects. Landsteiner and Popper injected the Old World monkeys with the spinal cord material. Both monkeys developed a disease that clinically and microscopically closely resembled that of the boy from whom the tissue was taken (14, 15). The ultimate irony came later. New World monkeys, like those forbidden to Landsteiner and Popper, are not susceptible to poliomyelitis, but Old World monkeys are. By a quirk of fate, these junior investigators became the first to isolate poliomyelitis virus from the nervous system tissue, then pass the virus into the appropriate experimental animal. Following up these observations, Landsteiner next showed that a virus caused poliomyelitis and that the virus infected the nervous system. In this way, an experimental model for the study of poliomyelitis became established.

In the following year, Landsteiner teamed up with Constantin Levaditi of the Pasteur Institute and reported the successful filtration of the material through a newer filter, the Berkefeld V type (16, 17). This established the final proof of the viral origin of poliomyelitis. Within several months, the scientific team of Landsteiner, Levaditi, and Mihail Pastia was able to detect poliovirus in organs other than the nervous system. They recovered virus from tonsils, membranes lining the throat, nasal secretions, and lymph nodes of the intestine taken from polio patients who had died. Results showing the viral cause of poliomyelitis were shortly confirmed by Simon Flexner and Paul Lewis at the Rockefeller Institute for Medical Research (18). Thus, by 1909, the groundwork was laid to develop a vaccine for poliomyelitis. The agent was known, tissues of the nervous system and other sites where the virus replicated were recorded, and an animal model was available. However, despite predictions in the early 1900s of the vaccine's imminent appearance, over forty-five years passed before an effective vaccine actually developed. The reasons

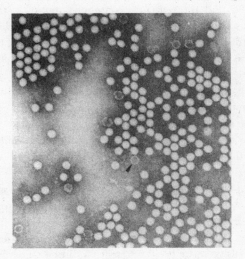

Figure 7.2 Electron photomicrograph of the virus that causes poliomyelitis. The arrow points to a particle that has no RNA genome (empty). The symmetrical icosahedral pattern is evident. Bar, 100 nm. Photomicrograph from E. L. Palmer and M. L. Martin, An Atlas of Mammalian Viruses (1982), courtesy of CRC Press, Inc.

were in some part the scientific complications still to be resolved, but in larger part the politics and scientific attitudes of those working on the problem.

The excitement created by Landsteiner's discoveries that a virus caused polio and that monkeys could be used for the necessary research offered the promise of controlling polio with a vaccine. At this time in 1909, Pasteur's earlier striking success in developing vaccines against a variety of infectious diseases of animals and humans was well known. Pasteur had established the principle of attenuation for fowl cholera and rabies. Further, the vaccine to control smallpox had proved successful and was widely used (see Chapter 4). With these events fresh in the minds of many, hopes of equal and rapid success for poliomyelitis were high. The time required to obtain such success was estimated to be short. The scientific mood was optimistic. In the spring of 1911, Simon Flexner at the Rockefeller Institute reported in the *New York Times*, "We have already discovered how to prevent the disease, and the achievement of a cure, I may conservedly say, it is not now far distant"(19).

When Flexner died in 1946, a vaccine against poliomyelitis was still far from being a reality. The long delay in producing a vaccine stemmed from a sad combination of circumstances. First, those who were making clinical observations of the disease were too widely separated from those working with the experimental model. This led to overemphasizing the leads obtained from experiments and not paying close enough attention to the actual course of poliomyelitis in patients. Although the Swedes had collected significant epidemiologic data indicating replication of virus in the gut and possible passage of the virus into the blood, this information was virtually ignored compared with the work of Americans primarily engaged in experimental research. The rhesus monkey preferentially replicated the virus in the respiratory area and not in lymphoid tissues of the gut, as patients did. Therefore, the experimentalists believed that the virus passed through nerves linking the respiratory tree to the brain. Second, it was not suspected until the late 1930s, and proven in the 1940s, that more than one poliomyelitis virus was capable of causing disease.

While in Australia, Macfarlane Burnet, who in 1960 was to receive the Nobel Prize in Medicine for his discovery of immunologic tolerance, became interested in Jean Macnamara's plan to evaluate serum obtained from convalescent poliomyelitis patients as a potential therapy for the disease. With that in mind, he began to compare the Rockefeller Institute standard strain MV with a recent isolate (the Melbourne strain):

We had two strains of virus, which in those days meant that we had in the refrigerator two sets of small bottles containing, in a preservative mixture of glycerine and saline, small pieces of spinal cord from monkeys that had been paralyzed by the appropriate type of virus. We knew that one of those pieces, ground up with saline, would give an extract capable of paralyzing the next monkey inoculated. One of these strains was isolated from a fatal case of polio in Melbourne, the other was obtained from the Rockefeller Institute and was a very virulent strain called MV. First experiments showed that the pooled convalescent serum could neutralize both viruses. Then Dame Jean [Jean Macnamara] and I found we had two monkeys that had been typically paralyzed but recovered, apart from their residual paralysis. One was paralyzed with the local strain, L, the other had been given MV with serum. The antibody had not been fully effective but the virus was weakened sufficiently to allow the monkey to survive. In order to obtain just a little more information, we tested them each with the opposite strain of virus. To our surprise, both were again paralyzed and died of polio. Recovery from infection with virus L therefore did not protect against MV nor previous infection with MV against L. We had only a few monkeys left but we were able to show that the two strains were antigenically different (20).

The impact of Burnet's finding was enormous, since an effective vaccine would need to contain the three strains of polio that were later identified.

But without a vaccine, without any control, poliomyelitis virus infection and the epidemics it caused struck terror in parents' hearts as each summer approached. Powerless to alter the progression of epidemics caused by the virus, state and local communities undertook quarantine measures in an attempt to isolate those undergoing acute infection from contact with susceptible individuals.

In New York in 1916 children were dying and being crippled from poliomyelitis virus infection. Many parents felt that sending their children to the hospital housing infected patients was tantamount to condemning them to death or being crippled for life. But regardless of parents' protests, some sick children were forcibly taken into isolation wards, initially by police officers (21). Nurses were soon substituted because they were more successful than the police in persuading parents to let their children go to the hospital. However, parental fears continued unabated. As reported by a social worker:

> The mothers are so afraid that most of them will not even let the children into the streets, and some will not even have a window open. In one house the only window was not only shut, but the cracks were stuffed with rags so that "the disease" could not come in. Babies had no clothes on, and were so

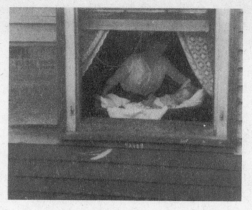

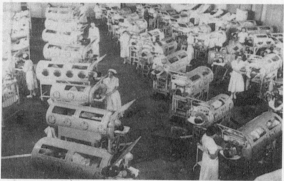

Figure 7.3 The concern and suffering from poliomyelitis are depicted in these two pictures. (Top) The isolation and forceable quarantine of a child newly infected with poliomyelitis during the 1916 epidemic in New York. (Bottom) Iron lungs were required to keep alive those with poliomyelitis infection involving nerves that controlled breathing. Without such temporary support many patients with paralysis of their respiratory muscles would have died.

wet and hot they looked as though they had been dipped in oil. I had to tell the mother I would get the Board of Health after her to make her open the window, and now if any of the children do get infantile paralysis she will feel that I killed them. I do not wonder they are afraid. I went to see one family about 4 p.m. Friday. The baby was not well and the doctor was coming. When I returned Monday morning there were three little hearses before the door; all her children had been swept away in that short time by the virus. The mothers are hiding their children rather than giving them up (22).

Under the sway of panic, people looked with skepticism and suspicion on government health offices. The selectmen of many villages, whose doctors were struggling with the impossible and failing to stop the epidemic or save patients from paralysis, resorted to homemade martial law. Movie theaters were closed to children under sixteen years of age. Swimming pools were closed. Children exposed to polio infection, or in an area where a case was found, were to be isolated for two weeks at home. Isolation could be best controlled in middle class and wealthy families, but poor children unable to be isolated were often forcibly taken to hospitals.

The 1916 panic precipitated by poliomyelitis virus infection in New York closely resembled the panic of yellow fever-stricken Memphis in 1878. On July 5, the *New York Times* depicted the wholesale exodus from the city of children of well-to-do. . . . 50,000 of them had been sent out of New York . . . to places considered safe by their parents. . . . Reports of persons fleeing from town continue to come in (23).

Similar to that earlier yellow fever exodus was the panicky response of several neighboring states and communities. The *New York Times* reporting on Hoboken, New Jersey, taking action against unwanted intruders stated:"Policemen were stationed at every entrance to the city—tube, train, ferry, road, and cowpath—with instructions to turn back every van, car, cart and person ladened with furniture and to instruct all comers that they would not be permitted under any circumstances to take up their residency in the city"(24).

In response to the continuing epidemic, Haven Emerson, the New York Commissioner of Health, announced on August 9 the postponement of the opening of New York City's public schools. As the summer continued, deputy sheriffs, hastily appointed, and some armed with shotguns, patrolled roads leading in and out of towns, grimly turning back all vehicles in which were found children under sixteen years of age. Railways refused tickets to those younger than sixteen. Ignorance, arrogance, and despair were evident. The notion was firmly held that below the magic age of sixteen there lurked the dread disease, whereas above it no menace existed either for the individual or the community.

But of course those over sixteen were not uniquely privileged to avoid poliomyelitis. Franklin D. Roosevelt, later President of the United States, was infected with the virus in his fortieth year:

I first had a chill in the evening which lasted practically all night. The following morning the muscles of the right knee appeared weak and by afternoon I was unable to support my weight on my right leg. That evening the left knee began to weaken also and by the following morning I was unable to stand up. This was accompanied by a continuing temperature of about 102° and I felt thoroughly achy all over. By the end of the third day practically all muscles from the chest down were involved. Above the chest the only symptom was a weakening of the two large thumb muscles making it impossible to write. There was no special pain along the spine and no rigidity of the neck (25).

As observed by his family, "Below his waist he cannot move at all. His legs have to be moved often as they ache when long in one position" (26).

The epidemics returned each summer and seemed to increase in severity. In Sweden it was reported that one of every five children who died succumbed to acute infectious poliomyelitis (3). Others were crippled. Not uncommon was the experience of Leonard Kriegel, who, while eleven years old and attending summer camp, shared a cabin with four other boys. Two of the four got poliomyelitis; one died and Leonard survived but was told he would never walk again without braces and crutches:

I started to scream and cry and bang my fists on the window, I remember. There was nobody in the house, thank God. But right after that I very methodically sat down and thought, "What do I have to do?" It was a month before my seventeenth birthday and I decided that what I had to do was to build up my arms. I realized I had to walk on my shoulders (21).

Josephine Walker also contracted poliomyelitis, the same year as Leonard Kriegen did. She was six years old at the time:

It was the most profound thing that happened in my young life. I remember the night I got sick. I remember my father returning from a business trip and coming up to say good-bye to me. I remember the ambulance coming and taking me off alone to the hospital. We were all put in quarantine for about two weeks, when nobody was allowed to see us.

My parents did everything for me that was needed physically—I was held and carried around by my mother for many years. They were in total denial about the fact that there was an emotional component to this. And so they pretended, after a while, like it didn't happen, other than the fact that I needed—you know—a little bit of medical help. People didn't talk about it; they didn't talk about the implications of it for my life. They just kind of let me go (21).

These stories were repeated many times throughout the world. No hope seemed in sight even though it was known that a virus caused the disease and

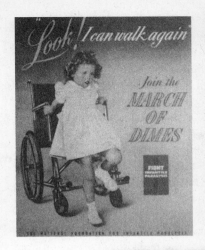
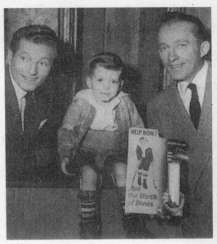
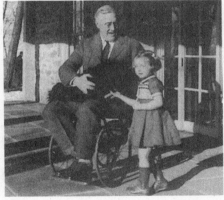

Figure 7.4 *The crusade to prevent poliomyelitis virus was initially organized by friends of Franklin Delano Roosevelt by the formation of the National Foundation for Infantile Paralysis. This organization sponsored the March of Dimes, a fundraising effort by mothers and other volunteers who walked city and rural neighborhoods and solicited funds at theaters and sports events. Fear of an illness that indiscriminately killed and crippled children brought together the diffuse fabric of American society.* (Top left) *One of the many influential posters dramatizing the issues to be addressed in the fight against poliomyelitis.* (Top right) *Hollywood stars Danny Kaye and Bing Crosby, who actively participated in the crusade.* (Bottom) *Franklin Delano Roosevelt and a child, both stricken with polio.*

that virus infection could, in some instances, be controlled through vaccination. A turning point finally came through the influence of Franklin D. Roosevelt, when his law partner Basil O'Connor and other associates committed time and resources to forming the National Foundation for Control of Infantile Poliomyelitis, dedicated to overcoming this disease. This organization publicized the effect of polio on children and with posters of crippled children induced masses of people throughout the United States to join a crusade of raising money toward seeking a cure. Similarly, the challenge to understand and prevent poliomyelitis attracted many dedicated scientists who sought to unravel the puzzle of its prevention.

A major factor delaying vaccine production was that a few authorities with political power essentially controlled the field and its scientific direction (2). Simon Flexner, director of the Rockefeller Institute, remained convinced throughout his life that poliovirus was exclusively neurotropic, that is, grew only in nerve cells of the brain and spinal canal. His rigidly held belief was that the virus causing poliomyelitis invaded the respiratory system and from there moved straight to the central nervous system. This view was in part based on study of the rhesus monkey, which is highly susceptible to infection with poliomyelitis but only by way of the respiratory system, and not the alimentary canal. With the prestige of the Rockefeller Institute behind him, Flexner's conviction became the prevalent, although wrong opinion, for many years. Unfortunately, the weight of esteem for Flexner and his followers successfully dampened, if not drowned out, the voices of Karl Kling and other Scandinavians whose systematic analysis of tissues obtained from humans dying of the disease enabled them to recover virus not only from the expected respiratory areas, in the pharynx and trachea, but also from the intestinal wall and intestinal contents. Kling and his group had also studied healthy carriers. They isolated poliomyelitis virus from the stools of healthy members of the families of patients with poliomyelitis virus infection as well as from other healthy individuals (27). But it was not until 1937–38 that Paul N. Trask finally confirmed the Swedish results. This evidence finally established without a doubt that poliomyelitis virus could reside in the intestinal tract, proof that Flexner had resisted for so long.

The agent causing polio is widespread and exists in most inhabited portions of the world. Usually the virus causes only a mild infection (98% to 99% incidence), a form that far outweighs the severe crippling disease that infects the nervous system (1% to 2% incidence) (28). The portal of entry of poliomyelitis virus is the alimentary tract via the mouth. The time from exposure to virus to the onset of disease is usually between seven and fourteen days but may range from two to thirty-five days. The virus likely binds to and enters through a special cell in the gut called the M cell. It travels from there to an area heavy in lymphoid tissues called Peyer's patches where it undergoes initial and continuing multiplication (28). It is this replication of the poliovirus in the lymphoid tissues of the gut that is responsible for passage of virus in the feces, which can subsequently contaminate swimming pools (or a city's water supply) and continue the cycle of infection. The oral route of transmission is likely responsible for the passage of poliomyelitis to susceptible adults who lack immunity to the virus but care for infants given the oral polio (living attenuated) virus vaccine. Although initially attenuated, the virus can revert genetically to a more virulent form during only a few days of replication in the infant's gut, thus leading to its presence in the infants' stools in their diapers.

The connection between spread of poliomyelitis in the summer and bathing in public swimming pools had been made by several public health officials earlier but never fully proved. For example, following the outbreak in Britain in 1911, a public health worker in London's East Side wrote in the *British Medical Journal*:

> I have for some considerable time interested myself in [bathing-water purification] at Poplar, where I have endeavored to give every bather a clean and sterile bath.
>
> I pointed out to the Baths and Waterhouses Committee of Poplar Borough Council the horrible dangers of public swimming baths, inter alia mentioning how quickly swimming-bath water changes its pristine sweetness even after being used only by a few bathers . . . and becomes after use by a number of bathers nothing more nor less than diluted sewage, and this condition exists often before the first day's use is finished. As it is during the months of July, August, and September that swimming baths are mostly used . . . it would possibly be of considerable interest to bacteriologists to take into consideration the possible connection of polluted swimming-bath water . . . and the disease and possible determination of one of the causes of poliomyelitis (29).

After infecting its victim, poliomyelitis virus is usually passed in stools for several weeks and is present in the gut and pharynx one to two weeks following infection. Undoubtedly the virus replicates in lymphoid tissues of the pharynx. Once this fact became known, it was apparent that the quarantine procedure was foolhardy, unless quarantine was kept in force for several weeks, during the time when poliovirus is being excreted (28).

Once the virus multiplies sufficiently in lymphoid tissues of the gut and pharynx, it travels into the blood and probably through nerve routes to reach the central nervous system. Poliomyelitis virus has been detected in the blood of patients with the mild abortive form (where no central nervous system illness is present) and also several days before obvious clinical signs of central nervous system involvement in patients who later develop either nonparalytic or paralytic poliomyelitis. The strategy of vaccination is to allow replication of the viruses in the alimentary and respiratory tracts, which stimulates an immune response and thereby prevents the transport of virus into the central nervous system.

Poliomyelitis virus infects only certain subsets of nerve cells and in the process of its multiplication damages or destroys these cells. The large so-called anterior horn cells of the spinal cord are the most prominently involved. Since these cells relay information that controls motor functions of the arms and legs, it is not surprising that poliomyelitis virus infection becomes visible as weakness of the limbs preceding paralysis. In severe cases, other neurons are involved including those of the brain stem where breathing and swallowing are controlled. Usually, though, the neurons in the cortex, the area of the brain associated with learning, are spared so that intelligence and cognitive functions remain intact. Fortunately, involvement of the lungs and throat was uncommon, even during the worst epidemics. When it occurred, it was necessary to place the patient in the infamous iron lung to force the exchange of air into and out of the lungs. Without such a device, death often occurred. If the paralyzed respiratory muscles recovered and the time in the iron lung was short, survival was possible.

The first mechanical respirator in wide usage was developed in 1929 by Philip Drinker, an engineer, and Louis Shaw, a physiologist working at the Harvard School of Public Health. Experimentally, air was pumped in and out of a box in which a cat whose respiratory muscles were paralyzed was kept alive. With commercial assistance, Drinker then constructed a man-sized respirator. The Drinker respirator, or iron lung, was a rigid cylinder in which the patient was placed, and at regular intervals negative and positive pressure was applied within the chamber. But during a severe epidemic of poliomyelitis in Copenhagen in 1952, with an attack rate of 238 polio patients per 100,000 individuals, the number of patients who could not breathe or swallow far exceeded the iron lungs available. This necessitated finding a more easily accessible and manageable solution. The approach was to apply the principles used in anesthesia of positive pressure ventilation—pumping air into the paralyzed lungs through a tube inserted directly in the trachea—essentially adapting a technique of the surgical operating room to the polio ward. The subsequently designed mechanical positive-pressure respirators eventually replaced the iron lung tanks.

By far the most common consequence of viral infection of humans is asymptomatic infection, usually a mild, short-lived disease. During this time, the virus can replicate and spread throughout a large population of hosts, for example, humans. Of those actually infected by the poliomyelitis virus, fewer than 1 to 2 percent become sick. The most common aftermath of such infection is that the patient develops fever, weakness, drowsiness, headache, nausea, vomiting, constipation, or sore throat in various combinations. These infected individuals recover within a few days. Alternatively, in a much smaller number of patients, stiffness and pain in the back of the neck are troubling for two to ten days, and in a small percentage, the disease advances to paralysis of the limbs and sometimes involves brain centers that control respiration.

The knowledge that poliomyelitis viruses infected the alimentary tract, and multiplied there before spreading into the nervous system, overcame a major stumbling block in controlling the disease. Yet two other barriers had to be removed before an effective vaccine was developed. The first involved the unusual complexity of poliomyelitis virus, compared, for example, with smallpox or yellow fever virus from which successful vaccines had been made. Immunity to smallpox or yellow fever was and is dependent on protection against a single virus strain. By contrast, poliomyelitis viruses are three distinctly different strains. Thus, any successful vaccine would need to include all these three strains. But this realization did not surface until the 1930s with the work of Macfarlane Burnet. Further, his discovery was not initially accepted. The painstaking work of the Typing Committee set up by the National Foundation for Infantile Paralysis in the United States by 1949 finally resolved the issue of the three polio strains, accomplished by typing over 195 strains of poliomyelitis virus isolates collected from near and far. These tests were done primarily on monkeys, because no one then had the ability to grow viruses in cultured cells. The second barrier was the actual production of a vaccine. The seminal contribution of Enders, Weller, and Robbins was their development of an easily manipulatable tissue culture system in which poliomyelitis virus could be grown (30). Finding that they need not use nerve cells, which are hard to manipulate and keep alive in culture, but could employ non-neuronal cells to replicate poliomyelitis virus, was the turning point in formulating their successful culture system and led to their Nobel Prize in 1956. Once these three conditions were met, it was possible to make a vaccine.

But which kind of vaccine was to be developed? Two approaches were considered. The first involved chemical inactivation of the virus. The idea was to purify the viruses grown in culture, then inactivate them with a chemical that would kill them thus destroying their virulence (ability to cause disease in a host) while retaining their antigenicity (the ability to generate an immune response). Objections to the chemical inactivation approach were several. One objection was that the inactivated virus would enter the body by needle into the skin and muscle, as opposed to the gut and alimentary tract. Because the virus normally enters its host through the mouth and digestive tract, providing live attenuated virus vaccine that mimicks the usual site of infection would be better for achieving optimal immunity. Further, attenuated live viruses had been the most universally successful vaccines, as witnessed by their ability to protect against smallpox and yellow fever. An additional argument was that, although the chemically inactivated vaccine might lead to immunity, this immunity was limited in time so that booster vaccinations would be required. Others argued that an infectious viral particle might escape the killing procedure and cause acute infection. This argument echoed a chemical inactivation approach that had been tried earlier. Maurice Brodie inactivated poliomyelitis virus by using formaldehyde. Soon afterward, in 1936, over 3000 children were inoculated with this chemically killed virus with tragic results: some of them developed paralytic polio (2). It was and is still not clear whether these incidents of polio resulted because no one knew at that time that the virus had three strains or because the virus was not sufficiently inactivated.

After discovery of the separate strains of poliomyelitis virus, the test of chemical inactivation was pursued in the early 1950s by Jonas Salk at the University of Pittsburgh (2,4,31,32). He successfully prepared a vaccine containing all three strains of poliomyelitis that had been killed with formaldehyde. To conduct the Herculean task of field testing the Salk vaccine, the National Foundation for Infantile Paralysis selected Thomas Francis, Jr., of the Rockefeller Institute. He organized and administered this study of 650,000 children, of whom 440,000 received the vaccine and 210,000 a placebo, all administered by needle inoculation. An additional 1,180,000 children served as unvaccinated controls. This clinical trial is still the largest in history.

Two years later, the Foundation's report indicated that the Salk vaccine was both safe and effective. It was at this announcement that the church bells pealed across the American landscape.

The vaccine was licensed several hours after the report. Yet difficulties remained. Although millions of dosages from five manufacturers licensed in the United States, Canada, and Denmark proved effective, with no hazardous effects, seven of seventeen lots made by Cutter Biologicals contained live, virulent viruses instead of killed viruses. This vaccine caused 204 cases of polio in which 75 percent, 153 of the recipients, were paralyzed and eleven died. The Cutter incident was a tragedy. What went wrong with their inactivation procedure was not clear. The results that followed were dramatic. Dr. Leonard Scheele, Surgeon General of the United States, withdrew the Cutter vaccine from the market. The Division of Biological Standards, located within at the National Institutes of Health (NIH), was created as a separate agency to ensure appropriate manufacturing standards and controls for medical compounds. Oveta Culp Hobby, Secretary of Health, Education and Welfare, resigned, although it was said for the purpose of spending more time with her family. Dr. William H. Sebrell, Jr., stepped down as director of the NIH and was replaced by Dr. James Shannon, who insisted on more effective safety measures. Dr. Victor Haase, director of the Allergy and Infectuous Disease Institute of the NIH where the Division of Biological Standards was formerly housed, also was replaced.

Yet the effectiveness of the Salk vaccine was evident. In the period of 1946 to 1955 preceding vaccination, the number of cases of poliomyelitis per year in the United States was 32,890 with 1,742 deaths. By contrast, after administration of the Salk vaccine, and before institution of the Sabin vaccine, the number of cases dropped to 5,749 with 268 deaths per year, although universal coverage for all susceptible individuals had not been achieved. In Sweden, where only the inactivated vaccine was and is used up to the present, poliomyelitis was eliminated.

Nevertheless, research on attenuated virus polio vaccines continued. Such attenuated viruses had been used for vaccination previously with dramatic effects. For example, Max Theiler had taken yellow fever virus, and passed it through animals and tissue culture to develop the 17D strain yellow fever vaccine, which was successful in the control of yellow fever. Theiler now began attenuation of poliomyelitis virus, showing in 1940 that Type II poliovirus of the Lansing strain passed through mice infected them but was not virulent for monkeys and presumably not virulent for humans. Interestingly, at the Rockefeller Foundation's Yellow Fever Laboratory in Brazil, Hilary Koprowski became aware of and impressed by Theiler's work on the attenuation of yellow fever virus. After Koprowski moved from Brazil to the United States and his job as Head of Research at Lederle Laboratories, he spent many hours discussing with Theiler the problem of immunization against poliomyelitis virus (6). From these discussions, he became convinced that the living attenuated vaccine would be the best choice. Beginning with Type II poliomyelitis virus, Koprowski adapted the virus to rats and then, in 1950–51, fed the resultant attenuated vaccine to twenty human volunteers (6). No side effects followed, and all those vaccinated made good antibody responses. These results, representing the first demonstration of the attenuation of a poliomyelitis virus and its success in immunization, were presented at a closed meeting called by the National Foundation for Infantile Paralysis (2,6). Koprowski next attenuated Type I poliovirus, again through passages in mice and rats, and eventually also

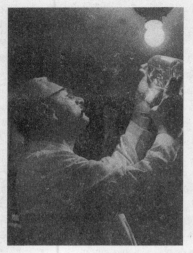 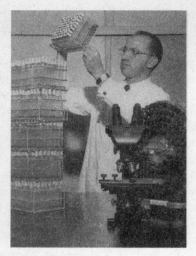

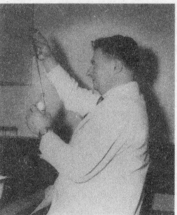

Figure 7.5 Three leading figures in the drive to make a vaccine to conquer poliomyelitis: (Top left) Albert Sabin, (top right) Jonas Salk, and (bottom) Hilary Koprowski. Salk worked on a chemically killed vaccine while Sabin and Koprowski worked independently on developing a living attenuated vaccine.

Type III virus. With the live attenuated viruses of all three types on hand, immunization trials were begun in 1956, with more than 1000 children vaccinated orally (6). Of those vaccinated, over 91 percent showed significant antibody responses to all three poliomyelitis virus types, and none of these children became sick with polio during subsequent epidemics. In 1956, Ghislain Courtois, director of the laboratory in Stanleyville, Belgian Congo, approached Koprowski about vaccinating chimpanzees in his chimpanzee camp. Later, when Courtois feared a poliomyelitis epidemic, he requested mass vaccination to local natives. In 1958, some 244,000 children of the Belgan Congo were vaccinated within six weeks and 67 percent achieved protection from the disease (2,5,6,31).

Independently, Albert Sabin began attenuation of the three poliomyelitis virus strains selected through tissue culture. By 1956 he had prepared a vaccine and had tested it in monkeys and in 113 human volunteers with excellent results (2,7,31,33). By then, Andre Lwoff at the Pasteur Institute showed that the best poliomyelitis virus variants were temperature-sensitive mutants selected from the now routine tissue cultures. The success of Lwoff and Koprowski spurred Sabin along in his quest for a more effective attenuated virus vaccine. By the end of the 1950s, the live attenuated polio virus had been clinically tested as an oral vaccine in numerous countries. The keystone of this effort was the successful mass vaccination of children in the USSR by Mikhail Petrovich Chumakov (2,7,31).

With completion of the main field trials and mass vaccination campaigns, all of which demonstrated both the safety and efficiency of oral poliomyelitis vaccine, it was time to decide which of the vaccines would be licensed. Accordingly, the U.S. Public Health Service called for the establishment of a committee to make that decision. That committee was composed primarily, but not exclusively, of scientists whose work was supported by the National Foundation for Infantile Paralysis. It seemed likely that the vaccine chosen would be a live attenuated one, and it would replace the chemically fixed Salk vaccine as the vaccine of choice. On August 24, 1960, the Surgeon General announced that the attenuated strains developed by Albert Sabin were recommended for licensing by authorities in the United States. Such a vaccine was easily administered, via a sugar cube, and could be given orally, the natural route by which poliomyelitis virus entered the body. This vaccine might best focus immunity locally in the alimentary canal where the virus attached to and entered M cells and then replicated in lymphoid cells. The attenuated live virus given as a vaccine at that site would then replicate and shed virus and viral variants, thereby allowing the immune system to be primed and to generate a diverse and protective immune response. Further, the vaccine had proven effective in massive field trials in Russia (2,7,31).

The committee decided on the attenuated strains developed by Albert Sabin over those by Hilary Koprowski. Overall, there seemed to be little difference between the two preparations, although several believed the Sabin vaccine slightly safer. Others suggested that the decision was based not on scientific facts or any advantage in one group of strains over another, but on political considerations (2,6). In his recent article on "A Visit to Ancient History" (6), Koprowski wrote that the decision was based simply on support for a member of the "coterie" as opposed to an outsider:

> My suspicion was confirmed at Christmas of the same year when Joseph Smadel, a member of the Committee, told one of my friends at a party that the Committee knew that there was no difference between the strains of all investigators but Sabin is an old boy and, since we decided only one set of attenuated strains will be licensed, we have chosen his strains.

John Paul, in his book, *A History of Poliomyelitis* (2), wrote:

> Koprowski remained one of the leaders, he was later to lament the fact that the vaccine against poliomyelitis which he had discovered should have been named the Sabin vaccine." Salk also saw himself . . . "as a young Turk fighting the establishment."

Such political positioning, disappointment, and resentment with the development of the poliomyelitis virus vaccine were no different than for the earlier smallpox and yellow fever vaccines. Benjamin Jesty and his supporters petitioned the House of Commons and the Royal Society to disallow Jenner's claim and substitute theirs in its place for the discovery of the smallpox vaccine. Wilbur Sawyer of the Rockefeller Institute never overcame his exclusion from the Nobel Prize awarded to Max Theiler for development of the yellow fever virus vaccine.

Regardless of whose poliomyelitis virus was chosen for the polio vaccine, all the personalities involved took great satisfaction when paralytic poliomyelitis was eliminated from Canada as well as North and South America by 1992. Moreover, at last count in 1996, the World Health Organization reported fewer than 2200 poliomyelitis cases per year for the first time since such epidemics were recorded in the nineteenth century. With the commitment of every country in the world, the eradication of poliomyelitis disease is planned for the year 2000, some 200 years after Jenner's description of the cowpox vaccine and the successful eradication of smallpox. In 1995–96 alone, over half of the world's children under five years, 400 million children, were immunized against poliovirus in the push to achieve global eradication by the beginning of the twenty-first century. We now understand that widespread vaccination of all susceptible persons is needed if the disease is to be eliminated.

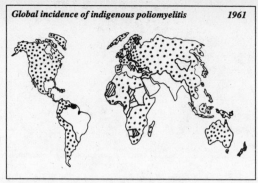

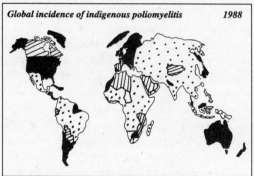

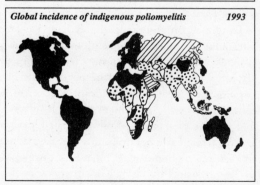

Figure 7.6 *The success of vaccination in controlling poliomyelitis.*
Incidence of indigenous poliomyelitis in 1961 (top), 1988 (center),
and 1993 (bottom). (Dotted areas) more than 10 cases; (hatched areas)
1–10 cases; (solid areas) 0 cases; (open areas) no report. The goal of
the World Health Organization is the total elimination of poliomyelitis
by the year 2000.

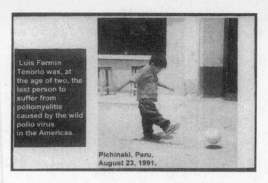

Luis Fermin Tenorio was, at the age of two, the last person to suffer from poliomyelitis caused by the wild polio virus in the Americas.

Pichinaki, Peru, August 23, 1991.

Figure 7.7 The last case of wild type poliomyelitis in the Americas.

Finally, the ascendance and contributions of Salk, Sabin, and Koprowski reflect an interesting change in biomedical research in the United States. Sabin and Koprowski came to the United States as immigrants, and Salk was the son of immigrants. All came from minority religious faiths that, prior to the 1940s and in some instances until the 1960s, had been largely excluded or under quota restriction from medical schools, residency programs, or work in premiere research institutes. The "Old Boys Club" lamented by Koprowski was already being dismantled at this time. Admission to join the great adventure of medical research was becoming available to those of talent, regardless of race, religion, sex, or national origin. Thus, the story of the conquest of poliomyelitis and the participation of Salk, Sabin, and Koprowski, in addition to recounting scientific accomplishment, also reflects a changing American culture and a continuing evolution toward a more democratic society.

Albert Sabin made many other significant contributions to virology. His work on sandfly fever, dengue fever, and herpes B virus, all preceding his study of poliomyelitis virus, produced significant discoveries. After the Sabin vaccine was licensed, he played a prominent role in its usage in many countries and devoted his energies in the Pan-American Union and the World Health Organization toward the control and eventual eradication of childhood illnesses in addition to poliomyelitis. Jonas Salk, throughout his life, continued to lobby for inclusion of his killed virus vaccine for usage in the United States. His vaccine is currently in use in Sweden, India, and several other countries. It is of interest that, after the deaths of Sabin and Salk, a program was proposed and recommended by the United States Commission in 1995, approved in 1996 by the American Academy of Pediatrics, and recommended in January 1997 by the Advisory Committee on Immunization Practices of the U.S. Department of Health and Human Services that gives both vaccines to an individual as a preferred course. By this scenario, the Salk vaccine is to be given early in life (to prevent attenuated virus-induced poliomyelitis while providing good neutralizing antibody titers) along with the Sabin vaccine that provides wider coverage, more lasting immunity, and both a humoral and cellular immune response. Hilary Koprowski went on to make major medical contributions to the development of the rabies vaccine, which is currently in use throughout the world. He also developed monoclonal antibodies to type and segregate individual strains of rabies arising in different geographic areas, and with his colleagues developed the first human monoclonal antibody for therapy of nonvaccinated individuals exposed to rabies.

PART THREE

PRESENT

AND FUTURE

CHALLENGES

CHAPTER 8

An Overview of Newly Emerging Viral Plagues

The Hemorrhagic Fevers

Lassa fever virus, Hantavirus, and Ebola virus—all equally lethal infectious agents but members of different viral families—share the ability to cause hemorrhagic fever (1). Once infected with any of these viruses, the victim soon suffers profuse breaks in small blood vessels, causing blood to ooze from the skin, mouth, and rectum. Internally, blood flows into the pleural cavity where the lungs are located, into the pericardial cavity surrounding the heart, into the abdomen, and into organs like the liver, kidney, heart, spleen, and lungs. Eventually, this uncontrolled bleeding causes prostration and death. We have no effective vaccine to prevent these potential plagues. Once hemorrhagic fever strikes, it is usually relentless and devastating.

The agents of hemorrhagic fevers can be placed into two groups. First are the killer viruses that are endemic in remote areas. These viruses await transport to introduce them into highly susceptible and distant urban populations. Representatives of this group are Lassa fever virus and Ebola virus, both of which are endemic in Africa. As in the sixteenth through nineteenth centuries when trans-oceanic ships brought not only goods to trade but also diseases like yellow fever, smallpox, and measles to infect residents of the New World (2), in the twentieth and twenty-first centuries airplanes provide transit for infectious agents. The only difference is that planes move viruses faster and further. Now a secluded individual incubating a potentially lethal infection, but showing no outward signs of illness, can quickly carry an infectious agent to the Americas, Europe, Asia, and Australia. The second virus group is endemic within the United States and is represented by Hantavirus. Although only a few hundred cases are known in several American states of the West, South, and North, the Hantavirus vector, the deer mouse, is found throughout the United States (1). Hantaviruses, like yellow fever viruses, are carried inside a nonhuman host. Hantaviruses aboard the deer mouse can be transported by this vector to cities and suburbs far from their customary habitat in much the same way that human travelers from tropical forests of the Americas or Africa, already infected but in the incubation stage, bring their diseases to other continents.

If a satisfactory vaccine were developed against these infectious agents, its greatest potential benefit would likely be in limiting the spread of the virus. Take measles virus as an example of controlling a highly infectious agent. Even with about 98 percent coverage by measles virus vaccine in the United States, a formidable number of persons remain susceptible to this infection (2% to 3% in a population of 260 million, or roughly five to eight million persons). Further, even though the measles virus vaccine is effective and efficient, the immunity it produces may wane two or so decades after vaccination, thereby adding to the number of individuals at risk. Travelers from an area where an epidemic of measles occurs, like Africa or Japan currently, may carry the incubating virus into the United States. In the event of outbreaks, massive vaccination of people in surrounding areas would likely be undertaken. With such blanket vaccination, virtually everyone would become immune, and the epidemic would be controlled.

Unfortunately for the victims of Lassa fever virus, Ebola virus, or Hantavirus, there is no vaccine to contain the diseases they cause. Even if there were, it is unlikely that the vaccine would be used in countries with a low incidence of these diseases. Nevertheless, the exotic viruses from Africa have made their way into the United States and elsewhere, although infrequently. So far, neither they nor the indigenous Hantavirus has caused a massive epidemic.

How do such new viruses surface? There are five major paths. First, viruses can modify their behavior and increase their virulence as they evolve through changes in their genetic material. Such genetic evolution can occur through reassorting of viral genes, recombination of a viral gene, or mutation within a viral gene. Reassorting occurs when a virus has multiple gene segments and swaps one or more of its segments with those from a different virus to form a new virus.

Studies in the laboratory show that a "new virus" created by such alterations can be much more virulent than the "parent" viruses, changing a mild and usually controlled infection into a lethal one. For example, a rodent virus, lymphocytic choriomeningitis virus, a member of the family that includes Lassa fever virus, contains two pieces of RNA (a so-called segmented virus). Each RNA piece contains two genes. The several strains of lymphocytic choriomeningitis virus are called Armstrong, Traub, or WE, named after their discoverers (Charles Armstrong and Eric Traub) or place of isolation (Walter and Eliza Hall Institute of Research, Australia); none of these strains causes disease when injected into two- to three-day-old mice of the Balb strain. Yet if the genes undergo reassorting so that the small RNA piece of Armstrong becomes joined to the larger RNA piece of Traub or WE, the newly generated Traub strain kills 88 percent of the mice, and the new WE strain kills all of them (3). There are many examples of viruses that swap segments of genes to become disease producers (4, 5). For humans, swapping of an influenza gene from birds or pigs with an influenza gene of man results in a new form of influenza virus that can wreak havoc on the human population (see Chapter 14) (6).

Another way in which viral genes change from a benign to a lethal form is recombination, the swapping of a gene within a single segment to form a new virus. Still another gene alteration process involves a single point mutation or several mutations during which just one or several amino acids replace those normally present and, thereby, create a new virus. The processes of reassortion, recombination, and single point mutation are shown in Figures 8.1 to 8.3.

Such point mutations usually occur once per 10,000 to 100,000 base replications with most RNA viruses like Lassa, Ebola, or Hanta. During continuous replication of viruses, a large population of mutants form that differ from their parent viruses. The few mutants that survive may grow better than the parent virus, may be attracted to and replicates in different cells, and may have greater disease-producing abilities.

The second way that new viruses surface is when their hosts undergo an increase in susceptibility to their harmful effects. This can occur via certain behavioral or social practices or through weakening of the immune system, for example, by taking immunosuppressive drugs.

The third route of viral emergence is when people increase their contact with vectors or humans that carry virulent viruses. As the need for more farming or grazing lands increase, humans penetrate the rain forests or enter

Reassorting (movement of whole gene[s])

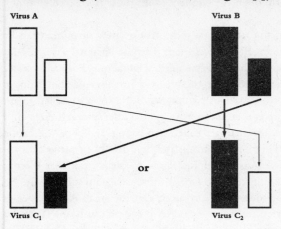

Figure 8.1 The reassortment of viral genes. Each of the boxes represents a separate piece of nucleic acid that may encode one or several genes.

Recombination (within a single gene)

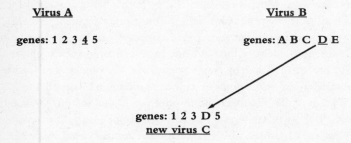

Figure 8.2 The recombination process. In this scenario, gene D from virus B replaces gene 4 of virus A to form new virus C.

new environmental niches and come in contact with rodents and other vectors that carry viruses. An example of behavior that encourages infection among humans is the African custom of staying in direct contact with sick relatives. In Zaire (renamed the Congo Republic in 1997), during the 1995 Ebola outbreak, healthy relatives shared hospital beds with the ill, and seventeen of the twenty-eight who had been healthy in one hospital contracted Ebola and died. In contrast, none of the seventy-eight persons who visited

Point mutation (change within a single gene)

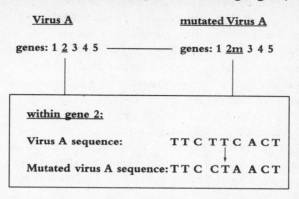

Virus A   mutated Virus A

genes: 1 2 3 4 5 ——————— genes: 1 2m 3 4 5

within gene 2:

Virus A sequence: T T C T T C A C T

Mutated virus A sequence: T T C C T A A C T

Figure 8.3 The generation of a new virus due to a mutation in a single nucleotide within a gene. Nucleotides depicted: (T) thymine; (C) cytosine; (A) adenine. Three nucleotides form (triplet) codons that encode specific amino acids. Amino acids are the building blocks to make proteins. The example shown is from real observations published from studies with lymphocytic choriomeningitis virus (7, 8). Virus A (which represents part of the sequence from Armstrong strain) has a mutation at base pair 855 of a T——►C. The TTC codon represents amino acid phenylalanine, while the mutated CTA codes for amino acid leucine. This single amino acid change allows the virus to infect adults, cause immunosuppression, and establish a persistent infection (CTA leucine). Upon infecting an adult host, the original virus (TTC——► phenylalanine) is cleared and neither persistent infection nor immunosuppression occurs.

Ebola patients in the hospital, but did not touch them or share their beds, got Ebola. A fairly recent modification in human behavior that has spread infection is the accessibility of rapid and frequent travel to distant areas.

The fourth origin of new viruses is simply an increase in their recognition and classification as biomedical and research technologies advance. For example, hepatitis viruses, which infect the liver, were categorized not long ago as hepatitis A virus, hepatitis B virus, and non-A/non-B hepatitis virus. With newer molecular techniques for identifying viruses by cloning, hepatitis viruses D through G have now been isolated, more than doubling just this one group of pathogens.

The fifth source of new viruses is referred to as the mystery source, because the cause is completely unknown. For example, the recent Ebola virus outbreak in Kikwit, Zaire, was traced to an index case, a charcoal worker/supplier. Before the outbreak was identified, he had infected thirteen of his relatives who also died. The social custom among his people of touching the dead was probably responsible for this instance of spreading infection. Those taken to the hospital infected hospital personnel and others, until the Ebola spread to 316 individuals, of whom 244 died. But how did the index case—the charcoal worker—get Ebola? Investigators are evaluating insects, rodents, other wild life, and so on, in concentric rings outward, like circles made when a stone drops in water, from the charcoal pit where he worked and the house where he lived. Still no clue has been found as to the origin of Ebola. In February 1996, thirteen individuals died in Gabon, West Africa, from Ebola after feasting on a chimpanzee. How the chimpanzee got Ebola is unknown.

The source of Ebola is not the only mystery involving newly emerging viruses. A new virus (morbillivirus), believed to be related to the measles family, caused an outbreak of acute respiratory disease in horses at a stable in Brisbane, Australia, in 1994. Then, two humans became infected, a stable hand who recovered after several weeks and a horse trainer who died one week after becoming ill. In 1995, a farmer in Queensland, Australia, died from a similar infection.

How many other mystery viruses will surface? How devastating will they be to humans? How do they form? This Pandora's box of mysteries and misery seems limitless. The historic struggle between viruses and humans described in the chapters on smallpox and measles and the more recent twentieth century battle with polio continues today and into the future.

Four of the best-studied, newly emerging viruses are the topics of the next four chapters. Of the first three, Lassa fever, Ebola, and Hantaviruses, relatively little is known except that they exist and can cause frightful disease. More is known about the fourth, HIV, but neither advice about its prevention nor current methods of treatment have yet significantly curbed its ever-rising death toll.

CHAPTER 9

LASSA FEVER

Lassa fever virus is a member of the arenavirus family (1). The name stems from *arenosus*—Latin for sandy—because of the characteristic fine granules seen by electron microscopy. Arenaviruses cause persistent infection in the host, that is, long-term infection that does not directly kill. Persistent infection, in general, does little harm to its animal host, because the two have evolved a near-symbiotic relationship, usually over the host's lifespan. The natural host of an arenavirus is often restricted to a single kind of rodent. The rodent host carries these viruses in its blood and passes them in its urine. It is by contact with such excretions from the rodent that humans become infected. Although no chronic or persistent arenavirus infections have been found in humans, Lassa fever virus has been isolated from the urine of patients as late as one month after the onset of acute disease. There are no known insects that transmit this disease. Consequently, spread to humans occurs only when humans come in close contact with the infected rodents in their natural habitat.

Lassa fever was first recognized in West Africa in 1969, but likely has existed in that region for much longer. The natural carrier is the rodent called *Mastomys natalensis* (multimammate mouse). In Africa, Lassa fever has struck natives, travelers on business, missionaries, and tourists. However, the cases that have provoked international fear are the several explosive hospital outbreaks. An example of the direct and continuous transmission of Lassa fever to five health care workers is the following initial report of the disease by John Frame and colleagues in 1970 (2–4):

Ms. Laura Wine, a nurse working in the small mission hospital, Church of the Brethren, in Lassa, Nigeria, was in good health until about January 12, 1969, when she complained of a backache. On January 20th, she reported a severe sore throat, but the physician found no signs to account for this on examination. The next day, she complained that she could hardly swallow; she had several small ulcers in her throat and mouth, an oral temperature of 100°F, and bleeding from body orifices and hospital-induced needle puncture wounds. By January 24th, she was suffering from sleepiness and some slurring of speech; late in the day she appeared increasingly drowsy. On January 25th, she was flown to Bingham Memorial Hospital in Jos, Nigeria. She died on January 26th after several convulsions.

A 45-year-old staff nurse, Ms. Charlotte Shaw, at the Bingham Memorial Hospital in Jos, Nigeria, was on night call when Ms. Wine was admitted on January 25th. Ms. Shaw had cut her finger earlier picking roses for another patient. As part of her nursing care, Ms. Shaw used a gauze dressing on her finger to clear secretions from the patient's mouth. She realized that there was a small cut on her finger and washed and applied antiseptic to the wound. Nine days later Ms. Shaw had a chill with headache, severe back and leg pains and mild sore throat, a clinical picture similar to that of Ms. Wine who died eight days earlier. Over the next days, Ms. Shaw had chills with fever to 102°–103°F, headache and occasional nausea. Seven days after the onset of symptoms a rash appeared on her face, neck and arms and spread to her trunk and thighs. The rash appeared to be petechiae (small hemorrhages) and blood was oozing from several areas of her body. Her temperature was 104.8°F. By February 12th, the patient's face was swollen; she had shortness of breath, a rapid, weak pulse . . . became cyanotic [bluish] . . . had a drop in blood pressure, and nurse Shaw died on the 11th day of illness. Autopsy showed the presence of fluids in each pleural (chest) cavity and in the abdomen. ,

A 52-year-old nurse, Ms. Lily Pinneo, working at the Bingham Memorial Hospital, Jos, Nigeria, had nursed both these patients and had assisted in autopsy of the second patient. She collected blood and tissue samples. On

February 20th she too developed a temperature of 100°F . . . followed two days later by weakness, headache, and nausea. Three days later she had a sore throat and petechiae and was admitted to the hospital. Since this was the third case in progression, the physician decided to send the patient to the United States for diagnosis and treatment. She was flown to Lagos, Nigeria, where she lay four days in an isolation shed and then to New York attended by a missionary nurse. . . . She was admitted to Columbia University Presbyterian Hospital (New York City) . . . was placed in isolation with full precautions attended.

Pinneo continued to be acutely ill with a temperature of 101.2°F. . . . The first night after admission, the temperature rose to 107°F. . . . She became extremely weak during the next six days. . . . Specimens from Ms. Pinneo were carried to the Rockefeller Foundation Arbovirus Laboratory at Yale for study. Meanwhile, over time the patient recovered strength slowly, became fever-free and was discharged from the hospital on the 3rd of May.

About one month later, Dr. Jordi Cassals of the Yale University Arbovirus Research Laboratory, who was working with specimens from Ms. Pinneo, felt unwell. Because he had developed symptoms like those of the other three patients, he was admitted to the Columbia University Presbyterian Hospital. The medical team decided to give the deteriorating Dr. Cassals blood from Ms. Pinneo, the blood containing antibodies to protect against Lassa fever. Within twenty-four hours, his temperature was normal. During his slow convalescence, virus was isolated from his urine. In keeping with the practice of arbovirology at the time, the virus was assigned a name from the first geographical community where it had been isolated—Lassa, after the area in Nigeria. Other tests confirmed that all four patients had been infected with Lassa fever virus.

A few months later, in the autumn of 1969, Dr. Cassals was well enough to resume his studies in the Yale Arbovirus Laboratory. By November work began on the live virus isolated from patients and passaged in mouse brains. Shortly thereafter, a laboratory technician, Juan Roman, near to but not in Dr. Cassals's laboratory, began to feel sick just before visiting his family in Pennsylvania. On the day after Thanksgiving, he entered a local hospital and died from Lassa fever before blood from an immune donor (such as Dr. Cassals or Ms. Pinneo) could be transfused. The Yale Arbovirus Laboratory decided not to perform any more experiments with live Lassa fever virus. The *New York Times, Time* magazine, and other publications reported that the virus was "too hot to handle."

Today in Africa, as in 1969, the scenario is that patients ill with fever of an unknown source are brought to medical stations or hospitals. Most are suspected of having malaria, a common disease accompanied by fever, or of having a bacterial or viral infection. Patients infected with the Lassa fever virus have a high temperature with throat and muscle pain. Invariably, their contact with the virus was as short as five or as long as twenty-one days earlier. After an additional week of progressively worsening sore throat, diarrhea, and cough, chest and abdominal pain appear. Frequently red lesions erupt inside the mouth; the patients become anxious and appear deathly ill as their faces swell and their eyes redden. Signs of blood leaking from small blood vessels, called capillaries, and from needle punctures made during hospital care become evident. As internal bleeding worsens, the patients become delirious or confused, and many convulse before dying.

Of African patients with Lassa fever, it is estimated that less than 10 percent appear at medical care stations; the vast majority stay in their homes or in the bush. Those who do come to medical clinics or hospitals, once they begin to bleed, have the potential to infect nurses, orderlies, and physicians through blood contamination, because their blood contains high levels of infectious virus. The death rate varies from outbreak to outbreak; the worst reported is about 60 percent and the least 10 percent. As the infection spreads, attending personnel and families of the patients sicken and die. Despite its virulence, Lassa fever has yielded but few of its secrets to those studying tissues from the victims. Little has been found to help in understanding the pathogenesis, or cause, of the disease (1). Although liver damage is the most consistent site of disease, only a modest number of liver cells are destroyed, probably accounting for the absence of jaundice in these patients. Damage to the spleen is common, as is the loss of white cells such as T lymphocytes and macrophages) in that organ. But many areas of the body become swollen, and, occasionally, T cells and other lymphocytes infiltrate a variety of tissues. The most significant fact is that so little tissue is actually destroyed—just enough to cause a lethal disease.

Could Lassa fever infection enter the United States unexpectedly? The answer is "Yes." In 1990, a resident of Chicago, Illinois, went to Nigeria to attend a family funeral. While in Ekpoma, Nigeria, he unknowingly became infected with Lassa fever virus. When he returned to his home in Chicago, he became sick and was admitted to the hospital for a fever of unknown origin. The specific cause of his illness was not diagnosed or understood during the short remainder of his life. He died of Lassa fever (5). Fortunately, the infection did not spread among the other hospital patients, the medical and technical staff, his friends, or family.

Currently, little research is under way in the West African countries where

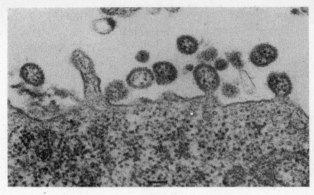

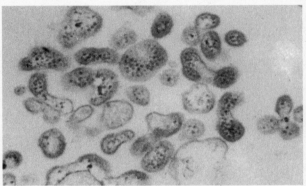

Figure 9.1 Lassa fever virus is a member of the arenavirus family. Virions are diagnostic because of the variation in size (polymorphism) and electron-dense ribosomes observed inside virions. The electron photomicrographs here are of lymphocytic choriomeningitis virus, a member of the arenavirus family that looks identical to Lassa fever virus. These related viruses are distinguishable on the basis of chemical, nucleic acid, and immunologic assays. (Top) Virus; (bottom) virus budding from cell. Both show the polymorphism and ribosomes.

Photomicrograph (top) from E. L. Palmer and M. L. Martin, An Atlas of Mammalian Viruses (1982), courtesy of CRC Press, Inc.; (bottom) courtesy of Peter W. Lampert and Michael B. A. Oldstone.

Lassa fever virus is endemic. Monitoring of the disease is virtually nonexistent, so understanding of its epidemiology and spread is limited. Yet the introduction of Lassa fever from Africa into Europe, the United States, and other densely populated countries remains a continuing concern.

CHAPTER 10

EBOLA

The Ebola virus first struck humans in northern Zaire (renamed in 1997 the Congo Republic). Of the 318 persons infected with Ebola virus in that outbreak of 1976, 88 percent died (1–3). The responsible strain of this virus, called Ebola Zaire, surfaced again a year later in southern Zaire, but only one person died. The virus then lay quiescent until 1995 when it erupted to cause the most recent epidemic in southern Zaire.

In that year, the world's attention focused on Kikwit, Zaire, whose population is approximately half a million. There Ebola virus is known to have infected 316 persons, and in its wake over 244, or 77 percent, died. But certainly the numbers were greater since no one could count individuals infected and dying in the bush. Most of those infected were young adults, on average about thirty-seven years old, although the range was from two to seventy-one years of age.

In the virus-stricken city of Kikwit, there was panic. The army sealed off roads and prevented anyone from leaving, a situation reminiscent of the yellow fever panic along the Mississippi River in Memphis 117 years earlier and of the barricades around parts of New York City 79 years earlier during the outbreak of poliomyelitis. Similarly, the Ebola virus began to move toward the city of Kinshasa, about 250 miles away from Kikwit, despite the blockades. Like the Ebola outbreak in 1976 in villages along the Ebola River 500 miles to the north of Kikwit, when nine of every ten residents who became infected died, Ebola virus again made its mark along the Kinshasa Highway.

At the beginning of May 1995, a large number of patients with hemorrhagic fever entered the hospital in Kikwit, Zaire. In short order, the patients hospitalized for treatment, the families accompanying them, and many nurses and doctors who treated these patients died of severe hemorrhages. Ebola was suspected by local physicians who had observed cases nineteen years earlier (2). As reported in the weekly magazine *Newsweek*** (4):

> When a 36-year-old lab technician known as Kinfumu checked into the general hospital in Kikwit, Zaire, last month, complaining of diarrhea and a fever, anyone could have mistaken his illness for the dysentery that was plaguing the city. Nurses, doctors and nuns did what they could to help the young man. They soon saw that his disease wasn't just dysentery. Blood began oozing from every orifice in his body. Within four days he was dead. By then the illness had all but liquefied his internal organs.
>
> That was just the beginning. The day Kinfumu died, a nurse and nun who cared for him fell ill. The nun was evacuated to another town 70 miles to the west where she died—but not until the contagion had spread to at least three of her fellow nuns. Two have since died. In Kikwit, the disease raged through the ranks of the hospital's staff. Inhabitants of the city began fleeing to neighboring villages. Some of the fugitives carried the deadly illness with them. Terrified health officials in Kikwit sent an urgent message to the World Health Organization. The Geneva-based group summoned expert help from around the globe: a team of experienced virus hunters composed of tropical-medicine specialists, microbiologists and other researchers. They grabbed their lab equipment and their bubble suits and clambered aboard transport planes headed for Kikwit.
>
> Except for a handful of patients too sick to run away, the hospital was almost abandoned when the experts arrived. While the team went to work, the Zairean government tried to cordon off the city to prevent more inhabitants from spreading the contagion across the countryside—possibly

---

even to the sprawling slums of Kinshasa, the capital, where most of its 4.5 million people live. The quarantine was mostly a hollow announcement; it's been years since there was a functioning government in Zaire. The international doctors sent people with bullhorns through the streets pleading with residents to stay home. And they managed to get a preliminary death toll—at least 58 of 76 confirmed sufferers had now died.

Specimens were collected and forwarded via the Belgian Embassy to the Institute of Tropical Medicine in Antwerp for evaluation. But they could not be tested there for diagnosis of Ebola, because that Institute no longer had the appropriate containment laboratory for such studies. In Belgium, as elsewhere including the United States, short-term political considerations had reduced funding for surveillance as well as research into infectious diseases. The samples then traveled from Antwerp to the Communicable Disease Center in Atlanta, Georgia, where tests proved that most of the patients were infected with Ebola virus.

At that time, public health officials sought travelers to Europe or other countries who had been in the Kikwit region during the time of the outbreak and who might be incubating the Ebola agent. One such family quarantined in England was front-page news. The quarantine lasted until blood samples could be obtained and analyzed to show that they were not carriers of the Ebola virus.

Undoubtedly, the reports of 280 cases of Ebola in Kikwit and its surrounding areas were gross underestimations of the true tragedy that had occurred. Why? First, the stigma of disease prevents many victims from coming into the city, so they die in their rural villages. Second, an epidemic is frequently under-reported or denied because of the fear that prospective tourists would cancel their visits. Zaire, like other African countries, depends on tourist travel for a major component of its budget. Nevertheless, teams of international scientists arrived and continue to search for plants, animals, or insects in which the virus might reside while not ravaging humans. So far they have turned up no leads.

Ebola virus can spread either through the air or by exposure to contaminated blood of infected humans. Relatives and family, who usually accompany African patients to the hospital and stay with them to administer nursing care, as well as medical and technical staff are at high risk of contamination by contacting blood or breathing infectious particles from these patients. The clinical course of Ebola virus infection is that of severe hemorrhagic fever (1). There is an incubation period, usually of six to ten days (ranging from two to twenty-one days), when the virus replicates in an infected individual. An

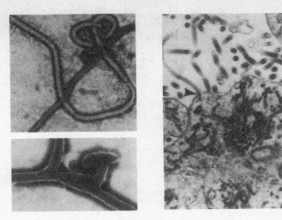

Figure 10.1 Ebola virus morphology. (Left) Electron photomicrograph of a specimen from cell (tissue culture) passage. Human blood specimen of the 1976 epidemic. (Top) Magnification, 35,000x; (bottom) magnification, 63,000x. (Right) Ebola virus (arrow) budding from the plasma membrane of an infected cell. Magnification, 28,000x. Pictures courtesy of Fields' Virology (Philadelphia: Lippincott-Raven, 1996).

abrupt onset of fever, frontal headache, weakness, muscle pain, slow heart rate, reddening of the eyes (conjunctivitis), and abdominal pain follow. Lethargy and lack of facial expression are common, with eyes having a sunken look. Two to three days later, the patients experience nausea, vomiting of blood, bloody diarrhea, and hemorrhage in the mouth and nasal passages, followed by prostration. A rash then appears, and death usually follows six to nine days after the symptoms start. For those few who survive, convalescence usually takes two to five weeks and is marked by profound exhaustion and weight loss. Spontaneous abortions are common consequences of this infection, and infants born of mothers dying of the infection become fatally infected.

Because the disease process moves with such rapidity and devastation, pathophysiologic changes have not been studied systematically (1). It is not clear how the terminal shock syndrome unfolds nor how the body chemistry makes holes in tiny blood vessels, causing the patients' profuse bleeding. There is no treatment for Ebola virus infection except rest, nourishment, and fluids. The only antiviral drug with potential benefits, ribavirin, has not been tested enough to evaluate its effectiveness.

Outbreaks of Ebola continue. A total of sixty cases with forty-five deaths (fatality rate 75%) occurred in the Gabon between mid-July 1996 and January 1997. Has Ebola escaped to the Western world? Again, yes. In 1989, in

Proven Filovirus Infections

Virus	Year	Location	Cases	% Mortality
Marburg	1967	Germany and Yugoslavia	31	23
Marburg	1975	Zimbabwe	3	33
Ebola (Zaire)	1976	Northern Zaire	318	88
Ebola (Sudan)	1976	Southern Sudan	284	53
Ebola (Sudan)	1976	England	1	0
Ebola (Zaire)	1977	Southern Zaire	1	100
Ebola (Sudan)	1979	Southern Sudan .	34	65
Marburg	1980	Kenya	2	50
Marburg	1987	Kenya	1	100
Ebola (Reston)	1989	Virginia, USA	4	0
Ebola (Reston)	1992	Siena, Italy	0	0
Ebola (Ivory Coast)	1994	Ivory Coast	1	0
Ebola (Zaire)	1995	Southern Zaire	316	77
Ebola (Zaire)	1996–97	Gabon	60	75

Data courtesy of Brian Mahy, Centers for Disease Control, Atlanta, Georgia.

Reston, Virginia, a suburb located less than twenty miles from Washington, D.C., at least four humans became infected during an outbreak of Ebola in monkeys. The infection caused by airborne Ebola virus was from cynomolgous monkeys brought from the Philippines (5). Of the 161 monkeys imported, more than half died over a two and a half month period. Luckily, and for unknown reasons, the virus failed to spread to other humans, even though the aerosol route of transmission was available.

Ebola virus is classified as a filovirus (*filo*, Latin for worm), because its structure seen under the electron microscope resembles that of a worm (1). Another member of that group of viruses is Marburg virus, which received its name after the virus caused an outbreak of infection in the city of Marburg, Germany. Unaware that monkeys carried Marburg virus, technicians and researchers used such monkeys as a source of tissue culture materials. At the initial outbreak in 1967, thirty-one persons came down with an acute illness and fever, and seven of them died before the virus was identified. The Marburg virus enjoys a near symbiotic relationship with the monkeys it infects, so does not harm them. But when man as an interloper comes into contact with fluids from an infected monkey, potentially fatal disease follows.

Ebola virus remains endemic in parts of Africa. Of over 4000 blood samples collected from individuals in central Africa, 24 percent revealed prior infection with Ebola. What its natural reservoir is, how it is transmitted, and where it lurks are all completely unknown.

Ebola—with its high fatality rate in humans, the lack of information about its natural history, origin of its periodic outbreaks, or mode of its transportation, and the inability to prevent or stop the disease once it begins—conjures up fears of a spreading disaster. These human responses to Ebola are reminiscent of events in the past associated with outbreaks of yellow fever and polio. The fear and fascination attached to Ebola outbreaks comes from our ignorance of how to treat, prevent, or contain the disease, and our helplessness in its wake.

CHAPTER 11

HANTAVIRUS

Hantaviruses are among the infectious agents currently found in the United States with the potential of causing a plague (1,2).

In 1993, a man and woman living on the Navajo Reservation in Muerto Canyon, New Mexico, suddenly experienced high fever, muscle pain, headache, and cough. Their lungs soon filled with fluid, and death from respiratory failure followed, first the woman and five days later the man. Public inquiries by the New Mexico Department of Health revealed twenty similar cases of acute respiratory distress in the region where the four states of New Mexico, Arizona, Utah, and Colorado join, the so-called "Four Corners" area. As with the initial two cases, all had been healthy young adults. Their mean age was thirty-four years. Of the twenty afflicted, half died.

Evaluation of these patients' medical histories and analysis of samples taken from their blood and tissues at autopsy by virologists at the Communicable Disease Center in Atlanta, Georgia, indicated that a common infectious agent

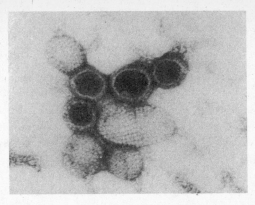

*Figure 11.1 Electron photomicrograph of Hantavirus. Magnification,
128,000x. Photomicrograph from E. L. Palmer and M. L. Martin,* An
Atlas of Mammalian Viruses *(1982), courtesy of CRC Press, Inc.*

was involved. This agent was identified as a Hantavirus (3), a member of the
Bunyaviridae family (4). Next, scientists using molecular techniques for study
of the virus's genes indicated that the Hantavirus recovered was quite different from previously isolated strains, all of which were known to cause hemorrhagic fevers and kidney disease, but not acute lung injury. The newly
observed disease was termed Hantavirus pulmonary syndrome (1–3). By
March 1995, some 106 cases of Hantavirus pulmonary syndrome had been
identified in twenty states and more than half of those afflicted died. Generally symptoms were fever, muscle pain, cough, nausea, vomiting, and headache
lasting about four but up to fifteen days and eventually requiring hospitalization. At admission, most patients were feverish with low blood pressure, and
low platelet counts (the cells required for clotting of blood), and had abnormalities (specifically, infiltrates) of the lungs visible in chest X-rays. Thereafter,
the patients developed pulmonary edemas, where the lungs progressively fill
with fluid. To this day, exactly how the virus causes disease is unknown; no
treatment other than supportive therapy and prevention are available. As in
Zaire and other sites of epidemics, the southwestern United States suffered
a decline in tourism once the outbreak of Hantavirus became public knowledge, causing economic hardship. Consequently, the original name of the
virus, Four Corners virus, was changed because of political and economic
considerations so that the virus is now called Sin Nombre virus, Spanish for
"no named virus" (1,5).

Hantavirus as a cause of hemorrhagic fever is not new (4). Evidence from
Chinese medical tests suggests its existence over 1000 years ago. In 1951–53

during the war in Korea, this virus made news with the outbreak of hemorrhagic fever in over 2000 United Nations troops. The transmissible nature of
the disease was first documented after serum and urine taken from patients,
then inoculated into human volunteers, produced the infection. Epidemiologic evidence suggested that wild rodents or ectoparasites carried the viral
agent, which in 1976 was identified in the lungs of field rodents in Korea.
Four years later the virus was isolated, grown in tissue culture, and used to
develop a diagnostic test. Although the virus is named for the Hantaan river in
Korea, Hantaviruses had infected victims in Japan, Russia, Sweden, Finland,
and several other European countries preceding the outbreak in the United
States.

The deer mouse (*Peromyscus maniculatus*), a natural carrier for Hantavirus,
was trapped and examined in the Four Corners area of the United States
(1,5). Later, several hundred of these rodents were trapped in other areas
where the Hantavirus pulmonary syndrome erupted, and the animals had
antibodies to the virus in their blood and also RNA sequences specific for
Hantavirus in their tissues. This viral RNA in the deer mice matched viral

Distribution* of Known Rodent Hosts
for Hantavirus and Location of HPS Cases,
as of May 17, 1995

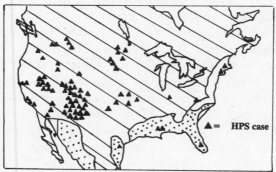

*Rodent distributions from: Burt WH, Grossenheider RP. *A Field
Guide to Mammals*, 3rd. ed. New York, New York. Houghton
Mifflin Company. 1980

*Figure 11.2 Known distribution in the United States of the
rodent vectors that carry Hantavirus and the location of human
cases of Hantavirus pulmonary syndrome. (Hatched area)*
Peromyscus maniculatus *(deer mouse); (dotted area)* Sigmodon
hispidus *(cottontail rat). Data courtesy of Brian Mahy, Centers for
Disease Control, Atlanta, Georgia.*

RNA sequences found in lungs of patients dying with disease. Clearly, the disease spread from the mice to humans interloping in their territory.

P. maniculatus rodents live throughout the North American continent from northern Canada to Mexico and across South America. These carriers of virus present a potential hazard to many large populations and probably have been responsible for cases of acute pulmonary disease occurring widely. Studies of *P. maniculatus* rodents outside the Four Corners region indicate that the Hantavirus carried by the deer mice is a newly mutated form. Additionally, several other rodent species also bear the virus. For example, investigation of Hantavirus pulmonary disease in a Florida resident led to the isolation of Hantavirus in *Sigmodan hispidus* (cotton tail) rats. Later a fatal case of Hantavirus pulmonary syndrome in Rhode Island was attributed to Hantavirus carried in the *P. leucopus* (white-footed) mouse. Similar isolates have been located in the northwestern part of the United States, in Canada, and as far south as Brazil. In only two years since its description in 1993, over 100 cases of Hantavirus pulmonary syndrome disease have been noted. The mortality rate is over 50 percent. The rodent populations widely ranging throughout the Americas capable of carrying Hantaviruses, coupled with humans at risk for exposure to such rodents in rural and urban areas, signal a potential health disaster. At present there is neither effective antiviral therapy nor vaccines available. The best strategy now is rodent control and avoidance of close contact with rodents or their excretions. But in winter, rodents frequently leave fields for the warmth of cities and their homes, possibly to deliver disease directly to our doorstep.

Lassa fever virus, Ebola virus, and Hantavirus, like other RNA viruses, frequently mutate. RNA viruses lack the fidelity that DNA viruses (such as smallpox) have to maintain stable genetic information of their nucleic acid structure. The enzyme (DNA polymerase) that makes DNA for DNA viruses is able to proofread what it has made. If a mistake occurs it corrects it. By contrast, the enzyme for RNA viruses (RNA polymerase) lacks this ability and is unable to correct errors. Consequently, RNA viruses have relatively high mutation rates because they lack good editing devices. Frequent and high levels of mutation for RNA viruses provides them with a greater potential for adaptability. Through a process of mutation and selection in a new host, more virulent or easily transmitted viruses may arise.

CHAPTER 12

HUMAN IMMUNODEFICIENCY VIRUS—"AIDS, THE CURRENT PLAGUE"

A plague as bad as any ever known now afflicts us, and the cause is a virus, the human immunodeficiency virus (HIV). The first description of HIV-infected patients appeared in the *New England Journal of Medicine* in 1981, in a paper that noted that four previously healthy homosexual men developed pneumonia from an infection caused by *Pneumocystis carinii* (1). The men also suffered fungal infections in the mouth and had multiple viral infections. This scenario of disease in persons with a low resistance to infection was consistent with the broad picture of an acquired deficiency of the immune system. The patients' infections by a variety of bacteria, fungi, and viruses produced prolonged fever and a marked reduction of cells now called the CD4$^+$ subset of T lymphocytes (1). Together, these observations suggested the immune system had broken down, and the cause was an infectious agent. The name "acquired immunodeficiency syndrome" (AIDS) designated this pervasive disease state. Reports now described hundreds of cases involving homosexual men, intra-

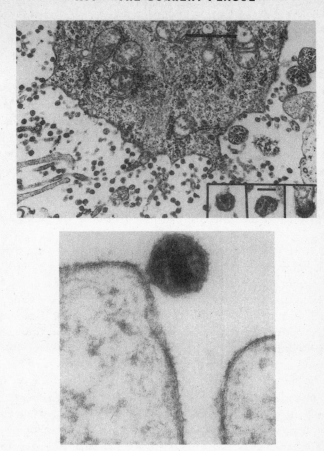

Figure 12.1 The virus that causes AIDS. (Top) *An infected CD4⁺ T lymphocyte that is producing virus. The insert is an enlargement of viral particles found in culture fluids. The virion is approximately 110 nm.* (Bottom) *The HIV budding from a cell's surface. Magnification, 180,000x. Note the bar in the virion that is characteristic of HIV. Photomicrographs courtesy of Robert Gallo.*

venous drug users, and others receiving blood products for medical therapy. By 1995, only fourteen years after the original report of the four AIDS patients, the Centers for Disease Control (CDC) and the World Health Organization (WHO) estimated that, in the United States, one of every seventy males and one of every 700 females were infected with the virus. As of October 31, 1995, a total of 501,310 persons with AIDS had been reported to the

CDC by state and territorial health departments; 311,381 (62%) had died. From 1993 through the present, among men that are twenty-five to forty-four years of age, AIDS is the leading cause of death, responsible for 23 percent of deaths. For women, it is the third leading cause of death (11% of all deaths) in this age group. These numbers are an underestimate of AIDS in the USA. Even worse, in Africa one of forty persons, both male and female, is infected. The incidence in Asia is not fully known but is expected to be astronomical. Estimates are that nearly 40 million individuals are already infected, with an expected 100 million to be infected by the end of the first decade of the twenty-first century. Although a few, scattered individuals have remained healthy for ten to fifteen years or more despite infection with HIV, to date not a single spontaneous cure of HIV infection has been confirmed. Those infected have either died eventually or have remained continually infected, waiting to die.

Infection by HIV is characterized by two major events. First, the victim makes a vigorous immune response against the virus (6). This is noted by the presence of antibodies to HIV (proteins in the blood that are induced by viral proteins (antigens) and react specifically with the inducing HIV proteins) and cytotoxic T lymphocytes (CTLs, cells responsible for cellular immunity). The CTLs arise during the early stage of infection and remain throughout its course (9,10) during which the patient is either clinically well or only minimally to moderately ill. The initial presence of CTLs directly correlates with a dramatic decrease in viral load; subsequently, the loss of CTL activity but retention of antibodies marks the phase of AIDS that culminates in terminal illness and death (9,10). Infectious virions and viral nucleic acid sequences are continuously present throughout the infection even in the face of a continuous anti-HIV immune response (6,9,11). Viruses or viral sequences are found primarily in monocytes and $CD4^+$ T cells in the blood (11,12), in lymphoid tissues (such as the spleen and lymph nodes) (12) as well as in microglia (13) (a form of macrophage) and endothelial cells of the brain (14,15) and other organs.

As the plague of AIDS continues and expands throughout the world, there is neither effective therapy for its permanent treatment and abatement nor is there a vaccine for its prevention. Treatment with the drug azidothymidine (Zidovudine) (AZT) or its counterparts, although effective in some instances, has at best worked only for the short term, presumably because of the rapid mutation rate of the virus and its ability to escape the drug's effects. The development of new drugs such as the HIV protease inhibitors offers the hope that combination drug treatment will remove the virus before HIV mutates and the virus escapes therapy. Whether HIV can be eradicated from an infected person and a case of AIDS cured is unknown. However, even with present combination therapy, nearly a quarter of treated individuals are not helped. The lack of a vaccine after years of research reflects how little is known about immunizing patients to protect them from an infectious agent that persists.

The virus usually enters the host in fluids (blood or semen) or within infected cells. The persistent infection that results remains intact in spite of an immune response whose products coexist with the virus. All the experiences with smallpox, yellow fever, measles, and poliomyelitis vaccines have focused on using an attenuated virus that could replicate in the host initially, would not harm the host, yet would provide enough stimulus for the host's immune system to combat and clear the viral infection. This experience has been useless for HIV. For reasons that are not yet clear but may reflect the victim's high level of viral load and unique properties of the virus, both the humoral (antibody) and cellular (CTL) arms of the immune system respond vigorously to HIV throughout the course of infection, yet some of the viruses remain in place. This situation is in stark contrast with viruses that cause an acute infection in which, if the infected individual survives, the immune response has cleansed viruses from all tissues. In this instance, viruses and the immune-response components coexist for but a short time (days), before either the virus or the immune response wins out. With HIV infection, both the virus and the immune response coexist but the duration can be years long—until the patient dies.

The discovery that HIV causes AIDS and is associated with cancer (Kaposi's sarcoma) has a long history. Nearly 100 years ago the search for a viral source of cancer began, and for the past thirty-five years the focus has been a specific viral group, the human retrovirus. Scientists now know that viral infections cause at least 20 percent of all cancers. Hepatitis B virus and hepatitis A and C viral infections are associated with liver cancer, Epstein-Barr virus infection with naso-pharyngeal cancer, papillomavirus with certain cervical and penile cancers, and HIV and herpes simplex virus-7 with Kaposi's sarcoma. Further, over one-quarter of the 600-plus known animal viruses have oncogenic potential, or the capacity to initiate in animals or cultured cells the kind of cellular division and growth that promote the development of tumors.

Transmission of cancers among animals had been attributed to viruses since the early part of the twentieth century. Many of these cancers arose from retroviruses, a family of viruses in which the replication of the viral nucleic acid is unique. By the rules of molecular biology, genetic information flows from DNA to RNA to protein. This is the pathway for DNA viruses like smallpox and for human genes. Other viruses contain their genetic knowledge in RNA (yellow fever, polio, measles, Lassa, Ebola, and Hanta are RNA viruses). They do not go through a DNA stage. However, unlike other RNA viruses, retroviruses essentially reverse the process, since their viral genetic material is RNA, but the RNA serves as a template (blueprint) for the synthesis of viral DNA through the action of a virus–specific enzyme, reverse transcriptase. This results initially in a DNA-RNA complex but the RNA piece is digested, leaving the DNA to carry out the replication process. In addition, the retrovirus DNA becomes integrated into the host DNA. With HIV, like all retroviruses, information goes from RNA to DNA to RNA to protein. To replicate in the host it infects, HIV must integrate its DNA into the DNA of host cells, a strategy that poses an extraordinarily difficult problem for the host's immune system in its effort to remove cells containing this foreign infectious agent.

A progression of events led to the concept that a virus could cause cancer. At the close of the nineteenth century, the first virus that infected animals had been reported by Froesch and Loeffler (15). By the first decade of the twentieth century, viruses were being isolated and manipulated as physical entities through the use of Pasteur-Chamberland-Berkefeld filters and experimental animals. It was during this time that the first retroviruses were shown to be transmissible agents that could cause cancers.

Vilhelm Ellermann and Oluf Bang (16), working in Copenhagen, Denmark, described the first true cell-free transmission of cancer. They showed that cancer induced by an agent "smaller than a bacterium," "an ultravisible [not seen by the microscope] virus," caused erythromyeloblastosis (a leukemia) in fowl. Filtered extracts of leukemic cells and blood transmitted the virus. However, at that time leukemia was not considered a cancer, and so this discovery lacked the impact of a later one. Another three years passed before Peyton Rous reproduced solid tumors (sarcomas) in fowls by injecting them with filtrates of a tumor obtained from a hen. At the Rockefeller Institute, Rous, after examining Plymouth rock hens brought to him by farmers, identified their malignant tumors as spindle cell sarcomas (17). He then demonstrated that these tumors could be transmitted to closely related animals. He prepared a cell-free, bacteria-free filtrate of such tumors and inoculated it into a healthy chicken; as a result an identical sarcoma grew in the second chicken (17). In the 1930s, breast carcinomas and other cancers were noted in mice. Active research on breast cancers transmitted from the mother to the offspring via breast milk focused on determining whether the cancer came from a virus as opposed to a milk factor. The research results showed conclusively that the cancer originated from a retrovirus, later called mammary tumor virus. Despite these accumulated findings that associated cancer with viruses, the investigations failed to achieve a major scientific impact. For example, when the National Cancer Institute of the United States was created in 1937, the committee of leading scientists who advised the newly created institute on "various lines of work which merit investigation" came to this conclusion regarding tumor virus research (18):

> It has been definitely shown that the animal parasites and bacteria which may incite malignancy in other organisms play no role in the continuation of the process [in humans]. The present evidence tends to indicate that the same may be true of viruses. As causes of the continuation of the malignant process, many microorganisms which may have been described as specific etiologic agents may be disregarded.

In spite of this advice, fifty years later the first human retroviruses were isolated by workers at the National Cancer Institute and shown to cause cancers (19,20).

From the 1950s through the 1970s, a plethora of discoveries were made regarding retroviruses. Many could cause tumors in mammals, and these could be transmitted vertically (into the fetus) as well as horizontally (from one individual to another after birth). In addition to their use of reverse transcriptase to begin replication from an RNA to a DNA, many but not all retroviruses infect cells of the immune system. Such infections often harm the immune system, most frequently by immunosuppression (suppressing its function). For example, a number of retroviruses can live in lymphocytes and macrophages and stop their activity as members of the immune system. Additionally, a new test was discovered to detect reverse transcription, effectively identifying retroviruses and facilitating study of retroviral infections.

The 1970s ushered in frantic activity by a large number of laboratories in the search for a retrovirus that could infect humans. Although many candidates were found, careful investigation showed that these retroviruses were not of human origin but rather were contaminants of non-human retroviruses. The most common examples were retroviruses that contaminated cells originally from subhuman primates or other mammals and used for culturing human materials. Another complication was the presence of host-dependent polymerases (enzymes important in making DNA) that, in many instances, were difficult to distinguish from the viral reverse transcriptase.

Many medical scientists are engaged in the current war against HIV. The two best known are Robert Gallo, formerly of the National Institutes of Health and later at the University of Maryland in Baltimore, and Luc Montagnier of the Pasteur Institute in Paris. Both of these investigators and the

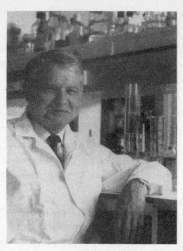

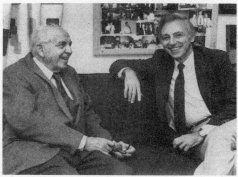

Figure 12.2 The two microbe hunters most identified with the isolation of HIV from patients with AIDS—Robert Gallo (bottom right) *and Luc Montagnier* (top). *Seated with Gallo is Ludwig Gross, a pioneer in the discovery of retroviruses in mice. The play between murine retroviruses and the lymphocytes they infect mimics many but not all the features of interactions between HIV and human lymphocytes. Photographs courtesy of Robert Gallo and Luc Montagnier.*

workers in their respective laboratories have been catalysts in the investigation of AIDS. However, as we will see, others have also played roles in establishing the importance of retroviral infections. As reflected in other chapters of this book, not one or two but many researchers contribute to defining and understanding each viral disease, as is true of HIV and AIDS. Many more will participate in its eventual control.

Robert Gallo was born and grew up in Waterbury, Connecticut. He was imprinted early in life by the sickness and death of his only sibling, his sister Judith, from leukemia at age seven (8): "I saw her emaciated, jaundiced, covered with bruises. . . . When she smiled I saw only caked blood over her teeth. . . . It was the last time [Gallo was 11] I would ever see Judy. . . . It remained the most powerful and frightening demon of my life."

This traumatic experience strongly influenced Gallo to choose a career devoted to understanding the biology of blood cells and leukemia. Initially, he trained in virology at the National Institutes of Health, where he became immersed in the study of retroviruses. As a result, his work joined together the fields of retrovirology and blood cell biology. Gallo's great contribution followed when he and his associates devised a method to grow lymphocytes (white blood cells) in culture and defined a growth factor required to maintain them (21). This, combined with a technique to detect viral reverse transcriptase developed by Howard Temin and David Baltimore, for which they shared a Nobel Prize in 1975, positioned Gallo to look for human retroviruses. First, tests had to be perfected that distinguished viral reverse transcriptase from cell reverse transcriptase. With such tests and the use of T-cell growth factor to grow lymphocytes from patients with leukemias, the first human retrovirus, HTLV-I, was identified from a patient with cutaneous T-cell lymphoma (19). Independently, investigators from Japan isolated a similar virus causing acute adult T-cell leukemia (22). One year later the second human retrovirus was isolated, HTLV-II, from a patient with hairy-cell leukemia (20).

The isolation of these first human retroviruses was made possible by finding reverse transcriptase activity in the fluid of cultured T cells taken from patients with leukemia. When Gallo and associates categorized the cancerous cells containing reverse transcriptase, by use of several techniques, the cells proved to be CD4$^+$ lymphocytes. Additionally, this reverse transcriptase was virus-specific, not a component of human cells, and was distinctly different from that of human DNA polymerase. Under an electron microscope the virus looked like a C-shaped particle, just like retroviruses found previously in non-human mammals. The genes of this virus were mapped and their relative positions to each other in the genome determined. A great many subsequent studies showed that HTLV-I was transmitted through blood products, during gestation from an infected mother to her fetus, and through sexual intercourse. HTLV-I, -II, and HIV are human retroviruses.

In December of 1981, Michael Gottlieb and colleagues in the Department of Medicine at the University of California, Los Angeles, examined four homosexual males who had been hospitalized for prolonged bouts of fever, and multiple bacterial, fungal, and viral infections—signs of a faulty immune system and low CD4$^+$ T-cell levels (1,5). All four patients developed *Pneumocystis carinii* pneumonia and one had a rare tumor, Kaposi's sarcoma:

> A 30-year-old previously healthy homosexual male (Patient 3) was admitted to the UCLA Medical Center with a one-month history of pain on swallowing, oral thrush [fungal infection], leukopenia [low peripheral blood white blood cell count] and a weight loss of 12 kilograms [about 26 pounds].
>
> Virus was not recovered from the initial biopsy sample. The patient was discharged . . . but readmitted five days later with fever, dyspnea [difficulty in breathing], and dry cough. . . . A chest film showed bilateral interstitial [lung] infiltration . . . biopsy specimen revealed abundant *Pneumocystis carinii*. . . . Cytomegalovirus was cultured from the urine [four months later] . . . the patient was readmitted [three months later] because of progressive cachexia (weakening and wasting). . . . A nodule which had not been present on previous examination was noted on the left wall of the chest . . . three similar lesions were located in the esophagus . . . biopsies revealed Kaposi's sarcoma.

Medical reports like this one of an acquired immunodeficiency syndrome with multiple infections and, sometimes, Kaposi's sarcoma soon appeared in numerous places (5). Clearly a new and dangerous disease had emerged not only in the United States but also in Europe and Haiti. Characterizations of patients from many medical centers all indicated a condition of prominent defects in the T lymphocyte arm of the immune system, especially the CD4$^+$ T cells, an association with pneumonia caused by *Pneumocystis carinii* bacteria, other infections, and, on occasion, the rare cancer Kaposi's sarcoma. The fatality rate exceeded 90 percent. Although the causative agent was not known, epidemiologic evidence suggested an infectious one, probably a virus.

This new disease became an epidemic by 1983. But how could such a disease suddenly appear? Past history with other infectious agents that have caused epidemics indicates that they frequently accompany major changes in social and/or economic conditions. The first epidemics of measles and smallpox infections likely developed as people left isolated villages and entered new, more densely populated cities along river basins. With measles, a new relationship between humans and the animals they domesticated probably also played a role, considering the similarity (amino acid sequence homology) between the human measles virus, the distemper virus of dogs (38% similarity), and the rinderpest virus of cattle (60% similarity). Migrations in ocean-crossing ships bore a clear-cut link with the initial epidemics of yellow fever in the New World. Still another factor was the exposure of remote populations to a novel infectious agent, for example, the natives of Fiji, who had never come in contact with measles virus, or the native American Indians, who lacked prior experience with smallpox and measles viruses. These populations were not only isolated but were relatively inbred so their gene pool lacked the extensive polymorphism of multiple genes seen in larger cosmopolitan areas. They would be more likely to possess "susceptibility" genes that had not been deleted (through deaths) owing to the lack of exposure to the specific infectious agent.

Probably in the 1960s or somewhat earlier, HIV evolved. Within a decade this new disease would reach epidemic proportions in parts of equatorial Africa. Before long, human infections with this new-found virus appeared in the United States, Europe, and Haiti. Likely contributing factors in the spread were the increase in international travel by airplane, increased promiscuity in sexual activity, especially with multiple partners, the increased use of blood and blood products for medical purposes, and, finally, the increase in intravenous drug usage.

Some believe that the source of this infection was a disease agent from subhuman primates that crossed species and entered humans. Perhaps a new virus then mutated or man became an interloper in a symbiotic relationship between a virus and a host animal. A second hypothesis is that a genetic change in an existing virus magnified its virulence and ability to cause disease. The third possibility is that humans became more susceptible than before to infection by HIV.

Reports of unexpected infections associated with pneumocystic pneumonia (bacteria), cytomegalovirus and other herpes viruses, and skin conditions related to Kaposi's sarcoma were becoming more prevalent by 1980–81. Physicians had observed similar infections earlier but usually in patients with suppressed immune systems. However, Kaposi's sarcoma had been extremely rare, and when it was observed, the usual victims were elderly men in and around the Mediterranean area or in Africa among Bantu tribes. By 1980, a few young males in the United States were afflicted with Kaposi's sarcoma and swollen lymph glands; instead of progressing slowly their cancers grew rapidly. The patients often proved to be homosexuals. But how to put the parts of the puzzle together?

The late 1970s and early 1980s was a dramatic period in the social acceptance of homosexuality. Initially hiding the truth of their sexual preference from themselves and others, gays started coming out of the closet and becoming politically active by the 1970s. They constituted a major voting block in San Francisco, comprising an estimated one in four registered voters and providing 70,000 votes in a city of 650,000. The promise of sexual freedom in San Francisco led to a migration of nearly 20,000 homosexual males to San Francisco from 1974 to 1978, with approximately 5,000 every year thereafter. An estimated 5 to 7 percent of the blood donated in San Francisco came from gays. HIV, the cause of AIDS, is found in blood, and soon cases of AIDS-like disease was being seen in transfused patients, children born of AIDS-infected mothers, patients undergoing surgical procedures, and hemophiliacs requiring regular blood transfusions or blood product therapy. Soon similar events were occurring in other large metropolitan cities harboring gays.

With social legitimacy came political and sexual freedom. Commercialization of gay sex spawned bath houses and sex clubs that soon became a $100 million business. With unlimited and unrestrained sexual freedom, regardless of gender preference, came blood diseases like hepatitis B, enteric diarrheal diseases like amebiasis and giardiasis, known sexually transmitted diseases like gonorrhea and syphilis, and pneumocystis pneumonia infections, Kaposi's sarcoma, lymphoid swelling, and fatigue. Although bath houses were breeding incubators for disease, few, if any, in the gay community seemed to care; few physicians, public health officers, politicians, or gay leaders were concerned. The first few random cases leading to the tidal wave of a full epidemic are described in a riveting story by Randy Shilts (23), then a reporter for the *San Francisco Chronicle*, who followed gay activities. His book *And the Band Played On* (23) chronicles the Castro Street happenings, the bath houses, and the beginning and relentless spread of the disease among a community and persons he knew:

> [T]he timing of this awareness [of the spread of AIDS] reflected the unalterable tragedy at the heart of the AIDS epidemic. By the time America paid attention to the disease, it was too late to do anything about it.
>
> From 1980 when the first isolated gay men began falling ill, years passed before all these institutions of public health, federal and private scientific research establishments, the mass media and the gay community leadership mobilized sufficiently to fight the disease.
>
> People died while the gay community leaders played politics with the disease, putting political dogma ahead of preservation of life. Local public health viewed the disease as a political problem.
>
> People died and nobody paid attention because the mass media did not like covering stories about homosexuals and several clergy, senators, congressmen, and leaders in the Reagan government saw it as a political and public relations problem that would not be supported by the majority of the voting public.

The HIV epidemic is unique. Unlike measles or smallpox infections, an acute illness after which either death or immunity result, HIV infection enables the viral genome to integrate into a host cell and cause persistent infection. Consequently, HIV infection most often progresses very slowly compared with the rapid infection of measles, smallpox, yellow fever, poliomyelitis, and the hemorrhagic viruses. Individuals are infected with HIV for many years, and each carrier has many opportunities to transmit the disease. Interestingly, HIV is poorly transmitted; only an estimated less than 5 percent of exposed humans are at risk of infection compared with measles and smallpox viruses, which infect greater than 99 percent of susceptible humans. However, one similarity between HIV and measles virus is that both viruses attack and infect cells of the immune system. The result is immunosuppression, leaving the victim at the whim of other infectious diseases, a situation called opportunistic infection. However, in the case of measles virus, the host immune system is able to overcome infection and clear the virus in the vast majority of cases. Exceptions are rare; as few as one in 100,000 to one in 1,000,000 individuals infected with measles virus develops a chronic disease called subacute sclerosing panencephalitis. In contrast, once it infects, HIV is unforgiving. The virus persists and few to no victims survive.

At first, HIV infection sets off a cascade of events that disseminates the virus to multiple lymphoid tissues. The immune response generated against HIV effectively lowers the host's viral load but does not remove all of it. The remaining viruses hide and cause a low-grade persistent infection. As the persistent viruses replicate, their offspring become trapped and/or infect a variety of lymphoid organs, causing chronic activation of cells of the immune system and secretion of products (cytokines) made by lymphocytes and macrophages. The cytokines activate other lymphoid cells, and virus replication accelerates until the ultimate destruction of lymphoid tissues results in AIDS—breakdown of the immune system. It is not clear whether the virus alone, or the virus in combination with an antiviral immune response (immunopathology), is responsible for disabling the lymphoid tissues and cells.

HIV was first defined as a clinical disease in American homosexuals living in or near New York City, San Francisco, and Los Angeles (5). The early symptoms are weakness, chills, enlarged and painful lymph glands, and, on occasion, purple skin blotches characteristic of the slowly progressive cancer (5,6) Kaposi's sarcoma. As HIV infection progresses, or even initially, effects on the brain become evident. Loss of concentration and poor mental function are common, especially with respect to solving puzzles or playing chess, which require a good attention span and ability to analyze new information. Many remain relatively healthy during the early phase of disease and may do so for several years. For others, death is rapid, in a single to a few years. The common thread for rapid progression of disease leading to death is the lowering of the CD4$^+$ T cell count usually below 100. Now AIDS has invaded the heterosexual community.

As new cases of AIDS increased to frightening proportions, scientists in several laboratories searched for the agent involved. Lessons learned from earlier work that led to the successful isolation of HTLV-I indicated the strategy to follow and the difficulties to avoid. First, cultured T cells from AIDS patients were grown with T-cell growth factor. Second, an assay for reverse transcriptase activity was needed that would be unique to this new human retrovirus and would exclude host DNA-dependent RNA polymerase or the previously described HTLV-I or -II.

In 1982 in France several scientists—mainly Jean Claude Chermann, Françoise Barré-Sinoussi, and Luc Montagnier—obtained lymph node tissue from an AIDS patient, Frederick B. (Bru HIV strain). They cultured lymphoid cells from this tissue, identified their content of viral reverse transcriptase, and infected healthy cells with materials from the culture. Chermann had been trained previously in the retrovirology of laboratory mice, and Barré-Sinoussi had experience in growing human T lymphocytes. Montagnier had worked with DNA viruses, interferons, and arenaviruses like lymphocytic choriomeningitis virus.

Simultaneously, in America at the National Institutes of Health (NIH), Robert Gallo had also obtained blood samples from patients with AIDS. Members of his laboratory had been the first to grow human T lymphocytes in culture using their newly discovered T-cell growth factor (21). They had also been involved in isolating the first human retrovirus, HTLV-1 (19,20). In 1982, they detected reverse transcriptase in lymphocytes from patients with AIDS.

These simultaneous research discoveries led to the back-to-back publication in 1983 by the French group (3) and the NIH group (2), both of whom presented data concerning the isolation of a retrovirus from patients with AIDS, and this virus's attack of T lymphocytes. In the same issue of the publication *Science* where these two articles appeared, Max Essex (4) and his colleagues in Boston reported on antibodies to cell membrane antigens that were associated with human T-cell virus in patients with AIDS.

Despite the excitement generated by these initial reports, several issues still needed sorting out. For example, it was not clear whether the newly isolated virus was a variant of HTLV or a separate and new human retrovirus. In the report by Essex (4), 35 percent of the blood samples obtained from AIDS patients also reacted with HTLV-I infected cells. Further, some of the virus particles seen by electron microscopy were interpreted by a panel of experts as being not a retrovirus but an arenavirus (8). However, subsequent studies rapidly and conclusively showed that this was indeed a new virus, now called HIV, not a variant of HTLV-I or II. The initial confusion occurred because some of the early cultures were infected with both HTLV and HIV (8). A characteristic profile of HIV soon became clear and ruled out an arenavirus as the agent of AIDS.

As recalled by one of the earliest workers on AIDS, Jean-Claude Gluckman (7):

I have been working on AIDS since the first case of the disease was diagnosed in France [December 1981]. . . . We adopted the hypothesis that the disease was caused by a retrovirus and defined what we considered to be the most propitious experimental conditions for the isolation of this hypothetical virus. Our idea was that the virus would be isolated more easily from patients with an AIDS-associated syndrome (essentially a generalized lymphadenopathy [enlargement of lymph nodes]) than from patients with AIDS itself. Because we thought it was likely that the lymph node hyperplasia was evidence of a localized immune response, which suggested the presence of a virus in the lymph nodes, we decided to search for the virus there, rather than in the peripheral blood of the patients. Rozenbaum and the virologist Françoise Brun-Vezinet contacted Luc Montagnier's group at the Institute Pasteur and brought them a lymph node specimen. That it was not a mere blood sample attests to the study group's contribution to the isolation of the virus. Montagnier, Jean-Claude Chermann, and Françoise Barré-Sinoussi went on to successfully isolate LAV, now known as HIV, early in 1983.

Robert Gallo (8) remembered:

Our earliest detections of reverse transcriptase [RT] activity in an AIDS patient dated to May 1982 with the cells of [patient] E.P. These cells were clearly positive for HTLV-I proteins (or very related proteins) and we worked on this isolation for a number of months. Our next set of detections occurred between November 1982 and February 1983, with at least five positives, but none of these samples were as vigorous as E.P. and most showed at best low level RT viral activity. Nevertheless, they appeared significant to us and they were negative for HTLV proteins; therefore they were suggestive of a new retrovirus. Our cell culturing was now speeding up . . . cells from both the symptomatic baby and the asymptomatic mother were positive for reverse transcriptase.

That was one of the earliest detections Phil[lip Markham] and Zaki [Salahuddin] [Gallo's associates] had and probably provided the first indication that the AIDS virus could, in fact, be transmitted either by intravenous drug abusers [the mother was a drug abuser] and/or by heterosexual routes, and also to babies of infected mothers. . . .

It was not until one year later, in 1984, when Gallo and his colleagues used a test they had developed to detect antibodies to HIV, along with epidemiologic data, that they firmly established HIV as the cause of AIDS.

Today we know that HIV has a narrow host range (6). It is a disease of humans, although certain subhuman primates can be infected by inoculation with either patients' tissues, cells infected in culture, or cell-free virus. Even before HIV was isolated, its routes of transmission in humans were well established (5). HIV enters its hosts by sexual transmission, transfusion of blood and blood products, and perinatal transmission from mother to fetus. The virus can travel during both homosexual and heterosexual activities, and, as with other sexually transmitted infections, the likelihood of infection is related to the number of sexual partners as well as to sites of sexual contact. In the United States, homosexual anal intercourse had been the major mode of transmission, whereas in Africa and the Caribbean, heterosexual vaginal intercourse appears to be the dominant mode. With the increasing incidence of HIV infection in American women, heterosexual intercourse has become a prominent means of infection that is predicted to increase dramatically. The virus can be isolated from semen and female genital secretions.

The HIV saga also mirrors social thought and conflicts of the 1980s and 1990s. Although HIV can pass through contact with contaminated blood or blood products, which involves a small but significant group of unfortunate individuals, the major route of transmission is sexual intercourse. Yet throughout the time since its discovery and to the present, in most instances HIV is one of the only sexually transmitted diseases that does not require reporting to health authorities in the United States. Due primarily to political considerations and unlike the sexually transmitted diseases gonorrhea and syphilis, HIV infection is rarely reported to local health boards by physicians nor are sexual partners informed that they are at risk for developing and spreading the disease. Further, in most states, blood tests for HIV infectivity are not mandatory to obtain a marriage license. However, those winds are changing direction. Beginning in January 1996, health care professionals in the state of California must provide information and counseling to patients receiving prenatal care. HIV antibody testing must be offered and recommended to the patient.

The principal source of HIV infection in newborns is infected mothers

(6). Although the virus can be transmitted across the placenta before birth, infection also occurs at the time of delivery through exposure to an infected genital tract or after birth through breastfeeding. An estimated 30 to 50 percent of infants become infected when the mother is an HIV carrier. Mothers requiring blood transfusions during delivery have been infected with HIV as have their babies.

Whole blood, blood cell components, plasma, and clotting factors have all been shown to transmit HIV infection. Even the transfusion of a single unit of blood from an HIV-infected person almost uniformly transmits HIV to the recipient. The spread of HIV through blood products is dramatic and tragic. For example, in Great Britain, roughly 6,287 hemophiliacs were registered between 1977 and 1991. During the period from 1979 to 1986, when blood products in Britain were contaminated by HIV, a total of 1,227 people were infected, or about one-fifth of those on the register. Because of the high degree of infectivity by HIV in blood products, undoubtedly about four-fifths of hemophiliacs who have not developed the disease received no contaminated blood. But because donated blood is often pooled, a single infected source has tainted other "clean" products. Therefore, ratios of infected to non-infected persons are at best very rough guides of the proportion of blood infected with the virus. In Japan half of the 4000 hemophiliacs developed HIV infection from contaminated blood products.

Fortunately, a test is now available to detect HIV in donated blood and has markedly reduced, although not eliminated, HIV transmission through transfusions in the United States and other industrialized countries. In the course of their research, Gallo and his associates developed this test to detect HIV contamination in blood as long ago as 1985. For the United States in 1984, a year before the test, 7200 people were infected with HIV through blood transfusions, compared to fewer than fifty people in 1996. Sadly, French health authorities purposely chose not to use this test, leading to the deaths of over 300 hemophiliacs and others transfused during surgery. Thousands more who became infected with HIV from that blood are likely to die. The delayed use of the "American" test in France evidently stemmed from two rationales. First, the French wanted to develop their own test and directly obtain the commercial benefits. Second, they wanted to sell blood products previously collected, since their loss might inhibit French dominance of the European blood product market (24). Subsequent investigations and criminal trials have led to the conviction and jailing of four health care workers. It still is not clear how high up in the French government the scandal goes.

Even worse, France was not alone. Similar events occurred in Japan and in Germany; large supplies of blood products collected for commercial use but not screened for HIV by the Gallo test were sold for profit. For example, currently Dr. Günter Kurt Eckert, the co-owner of the German drug laboratory Aproth, is on trial, charged with some 6000 counts of murder for selling blood products tainted with HIV. Elsewhere, other lawsuits have been settled and one is pending in which 300 HIV-infected hemophiliacs or their survivors contend that an American manufacturer continued marketing its blood-clotting products for two years after being informed in 1985 that the heating process used to treat the product would not kill the AIDS-causing virus. Economic and political considerations were more important to those in power and responsible for decisions in business and in government than the health of the public at large, their countrymen.

In February 1996, Health Minister Naoto Kan of Japan publicly apologized for the government's failure to prevent transfusion of HIV-infected blood in the 1980s. Even though officials learned of the risk in 1983, diseased blood was nevertheless used, causing about 2000 people to be infected. The consequences of a criminal investigation into this act led, in October 1996, to the arrest of Akihito Matsumara, who from 1984 to 1986 headed the Ministry of Health's Biologics and Antibiotics Division; of the two former presidents of Green Cross Corporation, the pharmaceutical house that had Japan's largest market share of blood products; and Takeshi Abe, former vice-president of Teikyo University, who was in charge of the AIDS study group that recommended the continued use by hemophiliacs of non-heated blood products in 1983. The charge is murder due to professional negligence resulting in death.

When scientific research approaches the borders of political debate and economic interests, the issue of who has access to data takes on critical dimensions. The potential for conflict over who best represents the public interest is clear when government controls accessibility to health care. That unfortunate issue has been played out with HIV and contaminated blood products in France and Germany as recorded here as well as in England with the possibility of contaminated beef causing a lethal degenerative disease of the brain, as discussed in the next Chapter.

Among the other sources of new HIV infections, intravenous drug usage bears a large and growing responsibility. In the United States it is estimated that approximately 25 percent of persons with HIV were once intravenous drug users.

Another important matter to be emphasized is routes that are *not* sources of HIV transmission. These include non-sexual personal contact, exposure to saliva (although virus has been reported in such fluids), exposure to urine, and exposure to insects. The paranoia that has occurred with the exclusion of HIV-infected individuals from school or business employment has no more logic than the blockades that were put up in 1916 by communities surrounding New York to prevent passage of poliomyelitis. Similarly, frightened people faced with smallpox or other epidemics who attributed the disease to unfavorable constellations of stars, to the wrath of supernatural powers, or to poisoning of wells by Jews or other ethnic minority groups sometimes paid for such superstitions with their lives. Even today, in our time of so-called enlightenment, some religious leaders, United States senators, and columnists who should know better have said that HIV infection represents the wrath of God on "unclean people." Ignorance is not a relic of times past but unfortunately still exists as does the frailty of humans faced with such catastrophic events.

AIDS is a true plague in our midst. Although the incidence of this disease is increasing, no therapy or vaccine is currently on hand. The resolution awaits newer methods of making vaccines that will arrest this disease. In the meantime, susceptible and exposed individuals throughout the world will continue to become infected, and if the expected trend continues, will die. Then the pool of persons who are susceptible—available to contract disease—will diminish. Perhaps a population resistant to HIV will emerge. Until we have better options, a few sensible measures would help to contain the AIDS epidemic. One option, quarantine, would be a fairly impractical, draconian approach for these patients, since it would require removal of infected persons for life. This "therapy," as far as is known, is currently being practiced in only one country, Cuba. More appropriate options are, first, screening of blood products and taking of detailed histories from blood donors, which along with HIV testing will protect the blood supply and make it safe. Second, and extremely important, limiting sexual intercourse with multiple partners and using safety-tested condoms would protect another large segment of potential victims. Third, ending intravenous drug usage will save lives for many reasons, only one of which is the risk of HIV infection. Last, a program that identifies those who carry the virus but does not interfere with their civil or economic liberty (which should be possible in an enlightened democratic society) would also slow the spread of this plague until an effective antiviral therapy and/or viral vaccine is found.

History teaches us that human ingenuity can overcome the most terrifying diseases. But, with evolution, many agents of diseases have become ever more complex or efficient, and new ones arise. For mankind to survive these calamities, the best efforts of scientists in medical research are required—not inhibited by political or religious interests, but supported by the full resources of governments and industry with conscientious participation by the general public worldwide.

CHAPTER 13

MAD COW DISEASE AND ENGLISHMEN

SPONGIFORM ENCEPHALOPATHIES—VIRUS OR PRION DISEASE?

Over 200 years ago farmers in England, Scotland, and France noted that some sheep suffered a progressive loss of balance, shaking, wasting, and severe itching that caused them to rub their hindquarters and flanks against any upright post. The name scrapie, or *tremblante* in France, was given to this disorder. Owners of healthy flocks recognized that their animals contracted scrapie only after introduction of new breeding stock later found to bear the disease. Eventually sheep exported from England infected herds in Australia, New Zealand, and South Africa. Only extermination of the affected animals stopped scrapie from spreading, but by then it was distributed widely throughout Europe, Asia, and America.

Nearly 100 years later, C. Besnoit (1) reported experimental transmission of the same disease by inoculating ewes with brain tissue from a sheep with scrapie. Then, in the 1930s, J. Cuillé (2,3) provided evidence for the first unequivocal transmission of scrapie to healthy sheep and documented that the agent was in brain extracts taken from scrapie-infected sheep and passed through filters with pores small enough to retain all microbes but viruses and perhaps other yet to be identified agents.

At about the same time and into the 1960s, a disease among the isolated Fore tribespeople in the central New Guinea highlands, an area under Australian administration, was investigated by Drs. Vincent Zigas and D. Carlton Gajdusek (4,5):

> In 1957, Dr. Vincent Zigas and I first described the rapidly fatal disease, kuru, a strong new subacute, familial, degenerative disease of the central nervous system (characterized by cerebellar ataxia and trembling) and restricted in occurrence to some 12,000 native Highland New Guineans of the Fore linguistic group, and to their immediate neighbors with whom they intermarry, and among whom it accounted for over half of all deaths.
>
> On first seeing kuru, we had suspected it to be a viral meningoencephalitis, only to find very little in the clinical picture, laboratory findings, or epidemiology to support such a suspicion, and nothing in the neuropathology to suggest acute infection. The epidemiological pattern of kuru occurrence suggested some genetic determinant of disease expression and this was supported by the restriction of the disease in peripheral areas to those individuals genetically related to the population in the center of the region.
>
> We were unable to demonstrate any contact infections in people living in close association to kuru victims throughout the course of their disease. We had early considered association of the disease with extensive cannibalism, but soon dismissed this as unlikely when cases of the disease were encountered in individuals whom we did not believe had engaged in the ritual cannibalistic consumption of diseased relatives, the prevailing practice in the region. The hypothesis that the disease might be an autosensitization, perhaps provoked by early sensitization to human brain through cannibalism in infancy or early childhood, likewise was not borne out either by neuropathology or by the search for autoimmune antibodies to brain antigen in serum specimens (6).

Kuru, which means shivering or trembling in the Fore language, was characterized primarily as a disease of women and children. Those afflicted had tremors, loss of balance, and an inability to form words, leading to a total loss of speech. Death followed usually in less than one year from the onset of obvious symptoms. This mysterious disease was confined to the highlands of New Guinea. The disease was common both in male and female children and in adult females, but rare in adult males. Anthropologic and epidemiologic investigations by Carlton Gajdusek suggested that the incubation period of this disease could be as long as thirty years or more. Even though he had first discounted the possibility, Gajdusek went on to record that the disease was transmitted by the practice of ritual cannibalism, a rite of mourning and respect for dead kinsman in which several tissues, including what we now know was highly infectious brain matter, were consumed by women and small children. Estimates indicate that over 90 percent of children and women partaking in cannibalism or smearing of their faces with diseased brain tissue developed kuru. Igor Klatzo, a pathologist at the National Institutes of Health in Bethesda, Maryland, who examined autopsied brains of kuru patients provided by Gajdusek, noted the punched-out Swiss-cheese appearance of the tissue and attributed it to the dropout loss of neurons. But what was the cause of kuru? A toxin? An ingredient in the diseased tissue? The answer was not clear, but an infectious agent, such as a virus, was low on the list of probabilities. Lack of the usual hallmarks of infection—that is, fever, malaise, rash, cough, and inflammatory cells in the fluids that bathe the brain—along with the unusually long incubation period, and, pathologically, the deficiency of inflammatory cells in the diseased brain—all spoke against a virus or any other ordinary infectious agent.

In those years nothing more than an educated guess linked kuru with scrapie. William Hadlow, a veterinary pathologist at the Rocky Mountain National Laboratory of the National Institutes of Health in Hamilton, Montana, entered the picture. His broad experience in natural scrapie infection of sheep led him to report that the brain injury in kuru reported by Klatzo and colleagues resembled what he had seen in animals with scrapie (7). Hadlow published his theory in the British journal *Lancet*, describing the resemblance between both disorders. Knowing that scrapie was transmissible, Gajdusek and his associate Joe Gibbs then promptly attempted to pass kuru to subhuman primates:

> In 1959, Hadlow brought to our attention the close similarities between the neuropathology, clinical symptoms, and epidemiology of kuru and of scrapie in sheep, a central nervous system degeneration known to be caused by a slow virus infection, susceptibility to which is genetically determined. Infection had before this seemed a very unlikely etiologic possibility for kuru. Now we were forced to reconsider the problem in the light of slow virus infections of the nervous system familiar to the veterinary virologists, of which scrapie and visna were the best elucidated examples.

With the realization that kuru (and possibly other degenerative diseases of the human central nervous system) possibly resulted from a slowly progress-

ing, long-lasting viral infection, Gajdusek realized that the laboratory procedures he and his colleagues had used earlier and which failed to uncover an
infectious agent were inappropriate. So in 1959 he resumed his search for a
transmissible agent in kuru but with a different strategy:

> The plan was for inoculation of unimpeachably adequate inoculum, i.e.,
> human brain biopsy material or very early autopsy specimens containing
> viable cells, inoculated without delay, or, if not so promptly inoculated,
> frozen promptly to -70°C in liquid nitrogen (dry ice) and inoculated at a
> later, more convenient time. The program was planned to include inocula-
> tion of many species of primates, including the chimpanzee, and long-term
> observation of these primates for, at least, 5 years after inoculation (6).

This procedure proved successful but, as suspected by Gajdusek, required
an incubation period of many months to several years. The next step was to
document continuous passage of the disease from one animal to others, and
this he did by using brains from ill or autopsied subhuman primates to infect
other subhuman primates. The results showed that scrapie and kuru were
much alike in their ability to transfer disease and cause destructive lesions in
the brain.

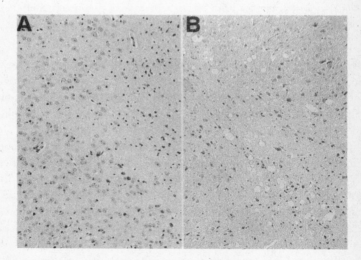

*Figure 13.1 Photomicrograph of a normal (A) and Swiss cheese-
appearing brain of a spongiform encephalopathy (B) that accompanies
human or animal disease. Photomicrographs taken from tissues studied by
the author.*

The pathologic similarity of kuru and scrapie to Creutzfeldt-Jakob disease (CJD), known previously as a chronic progressive dementia of humans tormented by tremors, led to the concept that a whole group of diseases involving slow progression and injury of nerve cells might be related. For his research on these lethal diseases called spongiform encephalopathies Gajdusek was awarded the Nobel Prize in 1976. As stated in his Nobel lecture on December 13, 1976:

> Kuru was the first chronic degenerative disease of man shown to be a slow virus infection, with incubation periods measured in years and with a progressive accumulative pathology always leading to death. This established that virus infections of man could, after long delay, produce chronic degenerative disease and disease with apparent heredofamilial patterns of occurrence, and with none of the inflammatory responses regularly associated with viral infections.
>
> Kuru has led us, however, to a more exciting frontier in microbiology than only the demonstration of a new mechanism of pathogenesis of infectious disease, namely the recognition of a new group of viruses possessing unconventional physical and chemical properties and biological behavior far different from those of any other group of microorganisms. However, these viruses still demonstrate sufficiently classical behavior of other infectious microbial agents for us to retain, perhaps with misgivings, the title of "viruses."

Related to scrapie, kuru, and CJD is a rare condition, the familial disease, Gerstmann–Sträussler Scheinker (GSS) syndrome. These patients have ataxia (the loss of coordination) and eventually develop dementia and die. The symptoms are similar for familial fatal insomnia, which presents itself as an inability to sleep that progresses to loss of coordination, dementia, and death.

In the laboratory, these diseases of sheep and humans were transmissible by feeding or inoculation, showed a similar pathologic picture, and had incubation periods varying from a few months to years, depending primarily on dose and strain of inoculum and genetics of the host. The infectious factor had at least one aspect of a virus, that is, it passed through filters small enough to retain all organisms except viruses, but it differed from viruses by virtue of its resistance to inactivation by treatments known to kill viruses such as boiling, application of 70 percent ethanol, ionizing and ultraviolet radiation, and the lack of an identifiable nucleic acid.

Unfortunate accidents have proven that such diseases are transmissible. For instance, transplantation of corneas from CJD patients or reuse of needle electrodes in neurosurgery has resulted in the passage of this disease from one human to another (8–10). Similarly, growth hormone used for medical purposes and extracted from pituitaries obtained at autopsies produced CJD due to contamination by tissue from patients whose CJD had not been diagnosed. Accidents of this kind are now largely eliminated: Corneas used for transplantation can be screened by careful history taking so that those obtained from diseased patients are not used; biotechnology companies now manufacture recombinant growth hormone so extraction from human tissues is no longer necessary; and electrode needles used to probe brain tissues are now disposable.

In 1985–86, bovine spongiform encephalopathy (BSE) in cattle was first identified in southern England, and within two years over 1000 cases surfaced in more than 200 herds (9). This was clearly a new disease in cattle, and by 1996 there have been over 160,000 confirmed cases in the U.K. affecting 59 percent of dairy herds as reported by the British Government's Ministry of Agriculture, Fisheries and Food. However, the data from 1988 to 1996 was sequestered by the British Government and denied to non-government independent researchers. When the information was finally available for analysis by others outside the Ministry, it was reported (11–13) that the number of sick cows was considerably higher than reported, or over 700,000.

Epidemiologic investigations indicated that the addition of meat and bone meal as a protein supplement to cattle feeds was the likely source of the infection. These studies also suggested that changes made in the rendering process during the early 1980s might be the cause. Why was the process changed? The high price and difficulty in buying oil because of OPEC policy and the Arab boycott were in part responsible. Suppliers who prepared the feed simply discontinued the use of petroleum-based products that inactivated disease agents. Thus sheep scrapie agent and/or possibly unrecognized BSE agents survived.

Epidemiologic studies indicated that the usual incubation period for cattle to develop the disease was four to five years, with a range of two and a half to over eight years. That interval coincides with the initial exposure of the cattle, presumably in the contaminated diet, from late 1979 through 1989, when this type of feed was banned in the United Kingdom. Even so, by 1993 cases of BSE, or mad cow disease, peaked at over 1000 per week (according to the Ministry of Agriculture, Fisheries and Food; these figures may be too low). There were 97,000 cases in Britain, 856 in northern Ireland, 37 in Switzerland, and five in France. Cattle exported from England carried mad cow disease to areas as distant as Arabia, the Falkland Islands, and Denmark. Presently reports cite about 300 cases per week.

In spite of the ban, according to the Ministry of Agriculture, Fisheries and Food, there have been over 26,000 cases of BSE in animals born after July 1988. Theoretically, these cattle should not have come in contact with contaminated feed. These findings suggest either that infected meat and bone meal is still entering the feeding process, although at a lower level, or that the disease may be transmitted horizontally and/or vertically (mother to baby) within herds.

In addition to controlling the BSE epidemic in cattle, measures were set up to gauge whether it was a human health problem and to safeguard the population from the potential risk of BSE transmission. As a defense measure, in 1990, a national CJD Surveillance Unit was established in the U.K. to monitor changes in the disease pattern of CJD that might indicate transmission of BSE to humans. The objective of this commission was to find out whether mad cow disease crossed species barriers to infect humans and manifested itself as CJD in people who had eaten infected beef and other cattle products (such as gelatin made from cattle bones) or had worked among diseased cows (e.g., dairy farmers, butchers, veterinarians). However, the long incubation period plus low incidence of CJD meant it might be many years before such surveillance yielded results.

A quicker route to obtain such answers seemed to be laboratory research. Since it was unethical to inject diseased cattle brains into humans, two alternative experimental approaches were taken to address the issue of whether mad cow disease might infect the human population. One approach was to take diseased cow brains and inoculate them into widely diverse types of sub-human primates. The second was to genetically alter mice so that they carried the human prion protein, a protein implicated in and necessary for development of the spongiform encephalopathies, and then challenge such mice with diseased cow brains. Both types of experiments take time, so a worried country could not even predict when to expect results. The U.K. held its breath, and, fortunately or not, the results soon arrived.

In 1993, the CJD Surveillance Unit reported that two dairy farmers who had been in contact with "mad cows" (with BSE) developed CJD. One was a sixty-one-year-old male who suffered progressive loss of memory, loss of balance, and inability to talk, then died within four months of the initial diagnosis (14). The second, a fifty-four-year-old male, also died within four months after a medical examination for rapidly progressing dementia, tremors, and ataxia (15). Both farmers had the classical pathologic lesions and abnormalities in prion proteins—key indicators of spongiform encephalopathies and now CJD.

But were these actually cases of mad cow disease transmitted to humans?

Although both dairy farmers had been exposed to mad cows and both displayed clinical courses and tests revealing CJD, they were only two of 120,000 individuals working in dairy farming and only two of about 51 million people in England and Wales where the expected incidence of new CJD cases is thirty per year.

Although CJD is the most common form of transmissible spongiform encephalopathies in humans, it is a rare disease with a uniform world incidence of about one case in two million persons per year. The disease most often strikes humans near age 65 (8–10) and is exceedingly rare before the age of thirty. Each year, approximately 85 percent of new cases appear randomly throughout the world and are of unknown cause, so are called sporadic CJD. The remaining 15 percent are either inherited associated with a mutation in the prion protein, or acquired. Examples of acquired CJD are from transplanted corneas, from cadaver tissues containing growth hormone, or, in the case of kuru among Fore tribesman, from cannibalism of diseased tissue. In the two dairy farmers, there was no history or biochemical evidence for inherited or acquired CJD. Further, no cluster of the disease followed among local butchers or veterinarians. So this chance finding probably reflected the rare cases of sporadic CJD that occur.

Then, in 1995, CJD surfaced in a fifty-four-year-old male dairy farmer in Britain with a three-month history of forgetfulness, altered behavior, slurred speech, difficulty in balance, and tremors (16). As this neurologic breakdown progressed relentlessly, analysis of his brain tissue led to a diagnosis of CJD. Again, since there was no evidence of familial or acquired disease, this case was considered to be sporadic CJD with no direct correlation to mad cow disease. At this time the European Committee Surveillance Project, while monitoring CJD in France, Germany, Italy, the Netherlands, and United Kingdom, found that the incidence of CJD in farmers closely approximated that in the general population and was not on the increase. So far, so good.

Unfortunately, this picture changed rapidly when, at the end of 1995, two additional cases of CJD emerged (17,18). The new complication was that the patients were sixteen- and eighteen-year-olds, not the usual sixty or so years of age. Previously, only four teenagers were known to develop CJD, a sixteen-year-old male in the United States in 1978, a nineteen-year-old female in France in 1982, a fourteen-year-old female born in England but living in Canada in 1988, and a nineteen-year-old female from Poland in 1991. No persons with CJD younger than thirty had been reported in the United Kingdom until these two.

The sixteen-year-old was a schoolgirl with worsening slurred speech, poor balance, and clumsiness. The eighteen-year-old boy's deteriorating memory showed up as a decline in school performance and an increase in confusion as his balance failed. Neither of these two teenagers had a history of familial dementia, and analysis of their brains failed to reveal the prion protein mutations that are associated with familial CJD.

Now the dilemma became acute. Was the world witnessing a new disease, perhaps associated with mad cow disease, or sporadic CJD? Both the small number of cases and the geographical separation suggested a sporadic nature; however, the patients' ages raised suspicion. As one might imagine, investigators considered the possibility that both patients had eaten contaminated beef or visited infected dairy farms.

Then one year later, in the first week of April 1996, the British journal *Lancet* published a report of not one or two, but ten cases of a new variant of CJD in the United Kingdom (19). These cases were unusual because of the patients' youth, ranging from nineteen to thirty-nine. All showed a relatively long duration of illness of fourteen months (average) compared with the average of four months for CJD. The brainwave features typical for CJD patients were missing, and the brain pathology revealed excessive amounts of abnormal prion protein lesions in the cerebrum and cerebellum, as opposed to the distribution found in older CJD patients in regions of the basal ganglia, thalamus, and hypothalamus. The brain pathologies of these recent cases were different from those of over 175 other patients with sporadic CJD. The CJD Surveillance Unit's proposal that Britain had a new variant of CJD ($_v$CJC) raised an immediate alarm that the affliction could be linked to mad cow disease.

Now a combination of fear and anger fed uncertainty (11–13,20–23). The resulting paranoia embarrassed the country's conservative government and is causing a huge economic loss (18) as hundreds of thousands of cows currently are being destroyed; several countries have already banned imports of British beef.

Is there or is there not a link between CJD and mad cow disease? Robert Will, a member of the British National CJD Surveillance Unit said, "I believe this is a new phenomenon." This was countered by the British government. Reassurance from the Prime Minister, the Health and Agricultural secretaries, the chief medical officer, and the Scientific Advisory Spongiform Encephalopathy Advisory Committee denied any increase in CJD or firm evidence that mad cow disease was transmissible to humans by eating British beef. However, John Pattison of the Advisory Committee said, "I would not feed [British] beef to my grandson."

The degree of danger, if any at all, could not be resolved with certainty because of the limited number of cases. With no reliable independent data available (11–13,20–23), public debate quickly focused on inadequate government handling of the situation and the manipulation of facts for political purposes. That is, as the accusations mounted, expert committees appointed by the government met in private, then uncovered evidence and reached conclusions that were made public only to the degree and with the bias agreed upon by officials. Two basic issues surfaced. The first was two-pronged: Who has access to the data and did government interests and the political spin it desired conflict with the release of scientific data? The second revolved around the balance between early release or publication of data speeding up the understanding of the disease and the concern that this information could create unnecessary panic if handled irresponsibly by the mass media.

The 1989 Southwood Report indicated that the incorporation of animal protein from sheep with scrapie into commercial cattle feed was the source of mad cow infection (9). The cause was changes in the preparation of cattle feed in the late 1970s and 1980s in the United Kingdom that allowed transmission of scrapie across species barriers into cows. With the banning of such feed in 1989, and the epidemiologic evidence that, if disease is transmitted across the species barrier from cows to man, there is likely to be an incubation period of three to ten or more years, then the 1996 cases represent only the tip of the iceberg. Because scrapie-contaminated feed was not banned until 1989, cases of CJD in the United Kingdom could be expected to increase markedly, perhaps into hundreds or thousands, for years to come. Alternatively, the CJD numbers may stay low, which would indicate a sporadic incidence of CJD and no relationship between the new CJD variant and mad cow disease. In a sense the experiment has been done with millions of people eating British beef from potentially spongiform encephalopathy-bearing cows from at least 1985, when the disease was first recognized, until 1989 at the earliest, when the ban on cattle feed was instituted or when subsequently infected cattle were removed from human food sources. The potential link between BSE and the new variant of CJD will be established or rejected by epidemiologic observations over the next ten years that chart new cases of the disease in humans. However, the fact that a variety of animals can develop spongiform encephalopathy after eating BSE-infected beef and the similarity in brain pathologies of BSE and the new CJD variant, different from the usual CJD-induced injury, are disturbing. Recently a twenty-six-year-old French man was diagnosed as having the variant of CJD, or vCJD. France has imported beef and live calves from Britain and BSE has been found in their herds.

A prion is a normal protein that, after modification, is associated with spongiform encephalopathic diseases like CJD and BSE. Prions are unique for each species so that human prions differ from cow or mouse, prions, for example. To study whether "material" in mad cow brain could modify human prions and cause disease, experiments were done in the laboratory where mice were genetically engineered to express normal human prion proteins and then given diseased cow brain. As yet, such mice have not developed any evidence of spongiform encephalopathy or CJD. However, mice as well as subhuman primates injected with similarly diseased brain tissue from cows did succumb to a CJD-like syndrome (22).

In evolutionary terms, the animal available for experimentation that closely resembles humans is the cynomolgus macaque monkey. These monkeys have prion proteins whose structures are 96 percent identical to human prion proteins. When such monkeys were inoculated with the new CJD agent or variant, the folded structure of their prion proteins changed in the same way the prion proteins in the British youths with the new type of CJD had changed (27). Then, when material from a cow with BSE was injected into the brains of three cynomolgus monkeys, two adults and one newborn, all three developed progressive central nervous system disease that included such abnormal behavior as depression, loss of balance, and shaking. These symptoms began within 150 days of inoculation and progressed in severity over the next ten to twenty-three weeks (24). After death, the autopsies of all three monkeys showed indications of spongiform encephalitis with special factors that more closely resembled brains from mad cows than brains of patients with sporadic CJD or cynomolgus monkeys given brain tissue from CJD patients. The startling similarity of the clinical, molecular, and neuropathologic features seen in these three cynomolgus monkeys with the CJD recently seen in young adults or juveniles in Britain suggests to some that the mad cow disease agent also caused the recent outbreak in humans. For other analysts, the association between mad cow disease and the new human cases is less clear. They support an alternative hypothesis that a new variant of CJD has occurred or been newly recognized because of enhanced awareness and focus on surveillance, and it is not related to BSE. Yet the recent finding that prion proteins show a characteristic chemical pattern (specifically, a high ratio of diglycosylated to unglycosylated forms) when obtained from BSE-infected brain tissue, brains of animals inoculated with BSE, and humans with the new CJD variant (25–27), a pattern opposite to that in sporadic CJD prions, suggests the relationship of these new human cases of CJD to BSE.

No one is sure whether the BSE agent fed to monkeys will cause disease, or, if it does, what amount is required and how long the incubation period will take. The most worrisome aspect is that, unlike spongiform encephalopathies in sheep, mice, and hamsters, for which there is no evidence for infection in humans, the similar agent in cows may well cross the species barrier and infect humans.

But what would constitute definitive evidence that BSE has spread to humans? The cynomolgus monkey experiments, the picture of nerve cell disease, the younger age of this new disease in humans, the fact that no vCJD has emerged in a country that does not have BSE, and the distinct chemical pattern that vCJD has unique strain characteristics distinct from other types of CJD, but similar to BSE, all evoke suspicion that a true epidemic rather than a false alarm may be on hand. The definitive experiments are in progress. That is, the incidence of CJD disease in Britain and elsewhere that does or, just as important, does not occur over the next several years in consumers of British beef from 1985 to 1996, especially before the banning of contaminated animal feed in 1989, should answer the question. An additional dilemma is that healthy sheep, pigs, and chickens have also been fed scrapie-contaminated products.

Confidence in the British beef industry cannot be restored by the scientific information currently available. The issue will be and has been, to a large extent, determined by the newspapers and the court of public opinion. On March 23, 1996, the (London) *Times* stated in a front-page article:

> The British beef industry was staring ruin in the face last night as the world boycott spread and the European Commission has declared the unilateral bans by 11 EU [European Union] countries legal. As prices continued to plummet at cattle markets, the Consumers' Association gave the starkest warning yet to stop eating beef and supermarkets urgently reviewed buying and labeling policies. MPs alarmed by the fallout from the admission that "mad cow" disease might have caused fatal brain illness in people have set up an inquiry into the handling of the affair and summoned ministers to give evidence next week.

On this same day *The Independent* headline read: "Should ours be the only children in the world to eat British beef?" It continued:

> The 13 scientists on the independent expert BSE Advisory Committee and CJD meet today at 11 am to ponder one of the most urgent questions ever to face the nation: is it safe for our children to eat beef? Nobody knows for certain if we are on the brink of an epidemic of CJD that could kill 500,000 people, or a containable problem that might claim a few score lives a year....
>
> With British beef now banned worldwide, and the Consumers' Association advising against eating it, we wait for the committee to advise ministers

on two crucial issues. Should parents ban their children from eating beef? And why might it be safe for adults to eat it but not children? Yesterday, Professor John Pattison, chairman of the committee, caused further confusion by saying that he would not feed beef to his three-month-old grandson who had never eaten meat but he would continue to give it to his nine-year-old granddaughter.

On March 24, the Sunday *Times* ran two front-page articles, one entitled "Scientists fear ban must now spread to lamb":

The safety of British lamb—so far untainted by BSE crisis—is in doubt as fears emerge that "mad cow" disease may have been passed on to some sheep. Although the government's scientific advisors admit they do not know the level of risk at present, they are considering taking the precaution of banning sheep offal. They argue that this would lessen the risk of the public being exposed to BSE agent from a second source. Such a ban would shatter confidence in British lamb, which has so far managed to escape the furor over beef.

The headline of the second front-page article read, "McDonald's suspends use of British beef in its burgers": "McDonald's is dropping British beef from its 660 restaurants in Britain from this morning because of the risks to customers from BSE, the company announced last night."

Further concerns arose when on July 18, 1997, the *St. Petersburg Times* reported: "St. Petersburg residents have just received another reason to stay awake at night worrying—the fear that the juicy steak they ate for dinner may have been contaminated with mad cow disease . . . meat (contaminated/banned British beef) was reportedly falsely labeled as Belgian, sold by the Belgian company Tragex-Gel to three French companies, imported into Russia and sold to companies in Moscow and St. Petersburg."

The problem is not just a British one. In September 1996, in an attempt to allay consumer and exporter fears concerning Swiss beef, a proposal reached the Swiss government to destroy 230,000 of its cows, thereby cutting the national herd by one-eighth but hoping to eliminate all traces of BSE. Currently, several countries including Germany and Austria have banned imports of Swiss beef and beef products.

What causes these spongiform encephalopathies? Originally the agent was thought to be a virus because of its unequivocal transmission of scrapie from sheep to sheep and then from sheep to mouse. Similarly, kuru and CJD have been transmitted to subhuman primates and spongiform encephalopathy from cow brains to mice, pigs, cats, marmosets, and healthy cattle. However, extensive scientific investigation has yet to identify the transmissible (infectious?) material (8–10).

Work pioneered by Stanley Prusiner (10) argued that it was not a virus but a modified host protein that caused spongiform encephalopathies:

> Based on these findings [the inability to detect nucleic acids in the infectious material, typical of viral infection], it seemed likely that the infectious pathogen capable of transmitting scrapie was neither a virus nor a viroid (viroids are small RNA nucleic acid molecules of unique structure that can replicate and cause disease (primarily of plants)). For this reason the term "prion" was introduced to distinguish the <u>pro</u>teinaceous <u>in</u>fectious particles that caused scrapie, CJD, GSS, and kuru from both viroids and viruses.

Experiments by Prusiner, Bruce Chesebro, and others have shown that, in the healthy brain, the prion protein exists in a form that is easily fragmented by certain proteolytic enzymes. In contrast, during the spongiform encephalitic disease state, the prion protein resists degradation by enzymes, leading to lesions in the brain. Consequently, many, but not all, researchers working on this problem believed that conversion from the susceptible (digested by enzyme) to the resistant (resists digestion) form of the protein is responsible for the disease (29). By this means, transmissible spongiform encephalopathies are spread by an agent that lacks information programmed by nucleic acids (as required for all viruses and other microbes) but is presumably programmed by a protein structure and is therefore unlike any other known agent of disease. Further, Prusiner and his colleagues as well as other scientists have learned that patients with inherited diseases of human nerve tissues like GSS syndrome possess a different (mutated) prion protein, unlike the prion protein present in the normal population. This prion-only hypothesis as a possible cause of spongiform encephalopathies is accepted by many, but not all. Others in medical science, for example, Chesebro, are not yet totally confident that a small virus or informational nucleic acid is excluded as the transmissible agent. At present an intense controversy rages among scientists engaged in one of the most interesting subjects in contemporary biology and biomedical research.

CHAPTER 14

INFLUENZA VIRUS, THE PLAGUE THAT MAY RETURN

In the spring of 1918, the German army again launched a massive attack on France, in anticipation of successfully concluding the First World War (1,2). Russia's withdrawal from the war enabled Germany to move more than one million experienced men and 3000 guns to the Western front, where Germany then had numerical superiority. The Germans placed thirty-seven infantry divisions there and had almost thirty more in reserve. This was the greatest assault force to date, and in several sectors it outnumbered those of the British and French by a ratio of four to one.

The French were desperate, and the British army had sustained serious losses at the battle of Passchendaele. With her enemies so depleted, Germany's main hope of success depended on an early attack, before additional American forces could arrive.

At first, the Germans made substantial progress, gaining over 1,250 square miles of French soil within four months. By May, the German army reached the Marne River, and its heavy artillery was within range of Paris. More than one million people fled Paris during the spring of 1918.

Everything seemed to be in Germany's favor, yet the very speed of her advance coupled with an outbreak of influenza virus infection brought her armies to near exhaustion. In late June, Eric von Ludendorff, the German commander, noted that over 2000 men in each division were suffering from influenza, that the supply system was breaking down, and that troops were underfed (2). Infection spread rapidly, and by late July Ludendorff blamed influenza for halting the German drive (2,3). Even as the German's strength began waning, that of the Allies was increasing. Americans continued entering France in numbers that replaced the great losses of the British and French. As the Allies reorganized, the French Marshal Ferdinand Foch took command. Foch and General Henri Philippe Pétain then led a grand offensive that aggressively blocked the German advance and regained French ground. The result led to the armistice that ended the war.

Even though the casualties, both military and civilian, were massive during World War I, deaths from the epidemic of influenza virus in 1918–19 surpassed the war's toll: Some 20 to 40 million people died of influenza in less than a year (3–6). This was two to four times the number of fatalities during the four years of war. It was estimated that one-fifth of the world's human population was infected, and 2 to 3 percent of those infected died. But this epidemic differed from all previous ones of its kind and those to come, because for the first time young, healthy adults succumbed. By contrast, in past and subsequent influenza epidemics, mostly the very young and the elderly died. Further, although respiratory infection was a common companion of influenza during the 1918–19 epidemic, pneumonia in young adults has been rare before and since. Over 80 percent of influenza-related deaths occur in people over the age of seventy who most often die from secondary bacterial infections. Yet the risk is almost as great for patients of any age who suffer from chronic heart, lung, kidney, or liver disease, for children with congenital abnormalities, or anyone undergoing transplant surgery or afflicted with AIDS.

The influenza pandemic of 1918–19 was lethal for healthy adults in the prime of life (3,7). The majority (nearly 80%) of United States Army war casualties were caused not by bullets, shells, or shrapnel but by influenza. From July 1917 to April 1919 this virus killed over 43,000 soldiers in the American Expeditionary Forces (7). In North America, the United States Bureau of Census recorded 548,452 deaths for the last four months of 1918 and the first six months of 1919 (4,7,8). In 1919 the American Medical Association reported that one-third of all deaths of physicians was caused by influenza-related pneumonia. Canada's death rate was proportionately high, with 43,000 deaths reported. In South and Central America, the devastation wrought by influenza virus was enormous. In the several Mexican states in which records were kept, over one-tenth of the population died; in Guatemala 43,000 deaths occurred in a total population of two million, and in Rio de Janeiro, with a population of 910,000, there were 15,000 deaths during the last three months of 1918. Chile lost 23,789 of her 3.6 million people in 1919.

Europe suffered as well; in England and Wales from June 1918 to May 1919, influenza killed 200,000, of which 184,000 were civilians. Ireland and Scotland lost approximately 20,000 each. Over the same time-frame in Denmark, with a population of slightly over three million, there was a mortality of 11,357, and Sweden, with a population of 5.9 million, had a mortality of 24,780. Prussia's seven million cases of influenza yielded 172,576 deaths. For the whole German population of over 60 million there were over 230,000 deaths, while France with a population of 36 million recorded nearly 200,000 civilian deaths. In the French army the mortality was three times higher than that reported for civilians.

In France, the American military forces taking part in the Meuse Argonne offensive of 1918 reported 69,000 sick with influenza. The infection was indiscriminate, afflicting soldiers, sailors, civilians, and leaders of many governments. Among the best-known were the Prime Minister of Germany, Prince Max of Baden; the Prime Minister of England, David Lloyd George; the Prime Minister of France, Georges Clemenceau; and Woodrow Wilson, President of the United States.

In Russia 450,000 lay dead from influenza and in Italy well over 500,000. Japan reported 257,000 deaths, but in no part of the world did influenza exact a more crushing toll than in the islands of the South Seas. In Western Samoa, the ship Talune from Auckland on November 7, 1918, introduced the disease into the islands of Upola and Savii. Within three months over 21 percent of the population died there and also in the Fiji islands and Tahiti. As one government official noted: "It was impossible to bury the dead. . . . Day and night trucks rumbled throughout the streets, filled with bodies for the constantly burning pyres." A British administrator traveling through villages in northern Persia noted that "in village after village there are no survivors."

The total world mortality for the 1918–19 influenza epidemic is not fully known (4,6,9). At that time a large part of the world's population, especially in Africa and Asia, was not tracked by adequate death records. Where records were kept, the lists for a period of less than a year indicated that over 20 million died. This figure can be extended two- to threefold if one extrapolates from subsequent records, providing an estimate of 40 to 50 million deaths.

Warren Vaughan of the Harvard Medical School, writing in the *American Journal of Epidemiology* in 1921, compared the mortality from influenza in the American army with that of other great plagues:

> This fatality has been unparalleled in recent times. The influenza epidemic of 1918 ranks well up with the epidemics famous in history. Epidemiologists have regarded the dissemination of cholera from the Broad Street well in London as a catastrophe. The typhoid epidemic of Plymouth, Pa., of 1885, is another illustration of the damage that can be done by epidemic disease once let loose. Yet the fatality from influenza and pneumonia at Camp Sherman was greater than either of these. Compared with epidemics for which we have fairly accurate statistics the death rate at Camp Sherman in the fall of 1918 is surpassed only by that of plague in London in 1665 and that of yellow fever in Philadelphia in 1793. The plague killed 14 per cent of London's population in seven months' time. Yellow fever destroyed 10 per cent of the population of Philadelphia in four months. In seven weeks influenza and pneumonia killed 3.1 per cent of the population at Camp Sherman. If we consider the time factor, these three instances are not unlike in their lethality. The plague killed 2 per cent of the population in a month, yellow fever 2.5 per cent, and influenza and pneumonia 1.9 per cent.

The influenza epidemic became known as Spanish influenza, not because the disease began in Spain, but because Spain, neutral during the First World War, had uncensored reporting of influenza's wildfire spread through its population: "The whole of Spain was invaded by a disease sudden in its appearance, brief in its course and subsiding without a trace." Influenza killed 170,000 people there.

This epidemic is believed to have reached Europe, Africa, and Asia via three major seaports: Freetown in Sierra Leone; Brest, France; and Boston, Massachusetts (8). Freetown was one of the major ports in West Africa and an important coaling station. There, local West Africans mixed with British, South African, East African, and Australian soldiers going to and coming back from the war in Europe. Over two-thirds of the native population of Sierra Leone came down with influenza, propelling the virus onto troop transports traveling back and forth to the war zone and eventually to the servicemen's home countries. Brest, France, was the chief disembarkation port for the European allies, and Boston was a main port for transporting U.S. troops to and from Europe. In Boston, within just a few days thousands became sick and hundreds died.

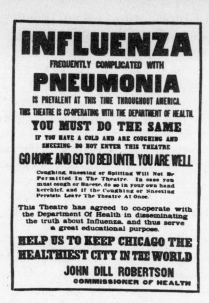

Figure 14.1 Poster warning about influenza pandemic, 1918–19.

Camp Devens, a U.S. Army camp, was located thirty miles west of Boston and housed 45,000 men. On September 14, 1918, thirty-six cases of influenza were reported, but by the end of September over 6000 had been infected, with sixty to ninety dying per day. One camp physician noted, "Bodies were stacked like cord wood." By the end of October there were 17,000 cases of flu, or one-third of the total population.

Within a month influenza spread from Boston to Philadelphia, where there were 700 deaths in a day, then to other parts of the United States. A common rhyme sung by young school girls jumping rope was:

> *I have a little bird and its name was Enza*
> *I opened the window and in-flew-Enza.*

Perhaps the spread of influenza is illustrated best by a study done in San Francisco. The first new case of influenza in 1919 appeared on September 23, brought by a traveler from Chicago. One month later, over 75 percent of nurses in San Francisco hospitals were sick, and all hospital beds were filled with those ill from influenza. Schools and places of public entertainment such as cinemas and theaters were closed by city decree. The city's Board of Supervisors ordered the wearing of gauze masks by the entire population. Everyone

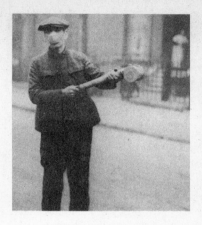 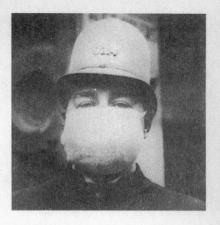

Figures 14.2 During the pandemic of 1918–19 buses and sometimes streets were sprayed with disinfectant to stop influenza (left) and police wore masks for their protection and to set an example (right).

who did not wear a mask paid fines or went to jail. On November 21 the sirens in the city shrieked to announce that masks could come off, but two weeks later the next wave of influenza began and struck 5000 in December alone. The wearing of masks again became mandatory. By February, when masks came off for the second time, over 3500 civilians had died.

Of course, public health officials attempted to deny suspected carriers of influenza entry to cities, as done for yellow fever, poliomyelitis, and Ebola. For example, J. W. Inches, Commissioner of Health of Detroit, notified commanders of all Army and Navy camps in the Midwest that Detroit, as of October 19, 1918, was off-limits to all military personnel except those in perfect health and traveling on necessary military business. They must carry a letter from a superior officer stating that these conditions were met, he decreed.

Just as the ships crossing on trade routes from Europe to the New World brought yellow fever, measles, and smallpox, so influenza traveled across the United States on routes once used by pioneers moving to the western United States. Railroad lines allowed the disease to move quickly to many localities, as did shipping lanes through the confluence of rivers and passage through mountain pathways. Influenza spread along the Appalachian mountains, the Great Lakes, the Santa Fe Trail, the inland waterways, the Mississippi River, and across the plains and Rockies to Los Angeles, San Francisco, and Seattle.

Italians introduced the term *influenza* in about 1500 for diseases attributed to the "influence" of the stars (4,6,8). Another possible origin is *influenza di freddo*, the influence of a cold. In the eighteenth century, the French coined the term *grippe* for the same symptoms. The disease can be present as an asymptomatic infection or as a primary pneumonia (3,6,9,10). Either way, it spreads from one individual to the next through the air in droplets launched by coughing or sneezing. Bringing individuals in close contact helps spread the infection, which in many instances initially travels among school children and from them to adults. Once exposed to the infectious agent, the victim incubates the virus for at least twenty-four hours and up to four or five days before the disease becomes obvious. The first signs are headache, chills, dry cough, fever, weakness, and loss of appetite. Generalized fatigue and, in some, bronchitis and pneumonia follow. In general, recovery to full strength following influenza viral infection may take several weeks or longer. Although influenza is a distinct and recognizable clinical entry, many patients and, unfortunately, some physicians, tend to group most respiratory ailments under a blanket term of "flu."

Although knowledge about the details of viral structure and behavior is recent history, as long ago as 412 B.C., Hippocrates described what seem to be influenza epidemics. Later, in Rome, Livy also mentioned the illness. From the Middle Ages, we have the following excerpt taken from a letter written by Lord Randolph in Edinburgh to Lord Cecil, dated 1562 (11,12):

Maye it please your Honor, immediately upon the Quene [Mary]'s arivall here, she fell acquainted with a new disease that is common in this towne, called here the newe acquayntance, which passed also throughe her whole courte, neither sparinge lordes, ladies nor damoysells not so much as ether Frenche or English. It ys a plague in their heades that have yt, and a sorenes

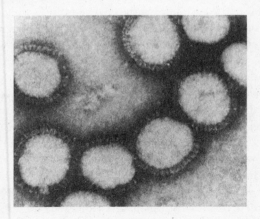

Figure 14.3 Photomicrograph of influenza viruses. Courtesy of
Fields' Virology *(Philadelphia: Lippincott-Raven, 1996).*

in their stomackes, with a great coughe, that remayneth with some longer, with others shorter tyme, as yt findeth apte bodies for the nature of the disease. The queen kept her bed six days. There was no appearance of danger, nor manie that die of the disease, excepte some olde folkes. My lord of Murraye is now presently in it, the lord of Lidlington hathe had it, and I am ashamed to say that I have byne free of it, seinge it seketh acquayntance at all men's handes (12,13).

Although suspected influenza epidemics occurred during several decades of the 1700s, Robert Johnson, a physician from Philadelphia, is generally credited with the first description of influenza during the 1793 epidemic (13–16). With his description available and improved public health statistics, epidemics were documented in 1833, 1837, 1847, 1889–90, and 1918.

However, the identity of the infectious agent that caused influenza remained debatable. In Germany, Richard Pfeiffer discovered "bacteria" present in great numbers in the throats and lungs of patients with influenza. Because of this agent's large size, it could not pass through a Pasteur-Chamberland type filter, causing many observers to speculate that influenza originated from a bacterium and not a virus.

Only by serendipity was the true nature of influenza as a virus discovered. This is a tale of pigs, hounds, foxes, and ferrets—all of which played decisive roles in the determination that influenza was a virus (17). This documentation for humans did not occur until 1933.

The story begins with J. S. Koen of Fort Dodge, Iowa, an inspector for the U.S. Bureau of Animal Industry. In 1918, he observed in pigs a disease that resembled the raging human influenza plague of 1918–19:

Last fall and winter we were confronted with a new condition, if not a new disease. I believe I have as much to support this diagnosis in pigs as the physicians have to support a similar diagnosis in man. The similarity of the epidemic among people and the epidemic among pigs was so close, the reports so frequent, that an outbreak in the family would be followed immediately by an outbreak among the hogs, and vice versa, as to present a most striking coincidence if not suggesting a close relation between the two conditions. It looked like "flu," and until proved it was not "flu," I shall stand by that diagnosis (18).

Koen's views were decidedly unpopular, especially among farmers raising pigs, who feared that customers would be put off from eating pork if such an association was made. Ten years later, in 1928, a group of research veterinarians in the U.S. Bureau of Animal Industry, led by C. N. McBryde, reported the successful transmission of influenza infection from pig to pig by taking mucus and tissue from the respiratory tracts of sick pigs and placing it into the noses of healthy pigs. However, these investigators were unable to transmit the disease after passing the material through a Pasteur-Chamberland type filter. Therefore, no evidence was yet available that a virus caused influenza. That situation changed when Richard Shope, working at the Rockefeller Institute of Comparative Pathology at Princeton, New Jersey, repeated McBryde's experiments within a year of the negative report. By reproducing influenza disease in healthy pigs by inoculating them with material taken from sick pigs and passed through the Pasteur-Chamberland filter (19–20), Shope provided the first evidence that viruses transmitted influenza of swine.

But was the influenza of humans like that of pigs? Did viruses cause both diseases? In the late 1800s and early 1900s, English country gentlemen and gentlewomen engaged in running hounds and hunting foxes became increasingly concerned over deaths of their dogs from distemper infection. The canine distemper virus, which is in the same family as measles virus, causes a respiratory disease often complicated by severe infection of the central nervous system that cripples and then kills dogs. Banding together and acting through *The Field Magazine*, a journal that catered to fox hunters, subscribers raised enough money to support research on canine distemper infection. Their efforts contributed to funding the Medical Research Council's (MRC's) acquisition of a farm at Mill Hill in north London, where the sick dogs could be isolated and studied. The pharmaceutical company Burroughs-Wellcome joined this effort to find a cure and to prevent the disease. Thus, in the 1900s those of sufficient wealth to afford fox hunting formed alliances with the government to set up the MRC and with a commercial company to find a vaccine. The alliance was successful; in 1928, the first vaccine became available to protect dogs from the canine distemper virus.

Initially, dogs were used for research on the virus and for studies to develop the vaccine, but problems soon surfaced. Among the difficulties were that some dogs had become immune because of a previous encounter with canine distemper virus, and that anti-vivisectionists and some pet owners objected to using "man's best friend" as a research tool. These problems vanished when ferrets were substituted for dogs. Hound keepers on the English country estates had noticed that ferrets also developed distemper, presumably transmitted from dogs. Soon ferrets replaced dogs in canine distemper studies in both the Wellcome and the MRC laboratories.

In 1933, the first epidemic of influenza since 1919 struck London and, as before, spread quickly. Among the many infected were several members of the

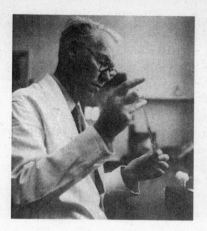
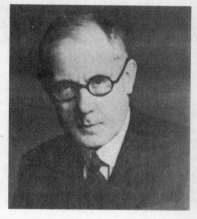

Figure 14.4 Sir Christopher Andrewes (left) *and Wilson Smith* (right),
*along with Patrick Laidlaw, were part of the team of medical researchers at
the Medical Research Council, Mill Hill, London, who isolated human
influenza virus.*

research staff at Wellcome and MRC laboratories. However, unexpectedly,
ferrets kept at the Wellcome laboratory also became ill, with symptoms of
wheezing, sneezing, and coughing reminiscent of human influenza infection.
When Wilson Smith, a senior researcher at the MRC unit, recognized the situation, he infected ferrets with nasal washings from influenza-infected
patients. As the ferrets came down with the influenza-like syndrome, both
Smith and Christopher Andrewes examined them. A few days later, Andrewes
came down with influenza. Smith obtained washings from Andrewes's throat,
passed the material through a Pasteur-Chamberland-like filter, then injected
the filtrate into healthy ferrets. Soon they too evidenced sneezing and coughing along with a discharge from the nose and eyes and a raised temperature.
Here was the first evidence that a virus caused human influenza, which at the
same time fulfilled Koch's postulates (21).

Following his studies with tuberculosis, Robert Koch formalized the crite-
ria eventually called Koch's postulates to distinguish a microbe-causing disease
from one that is a happenstance passenger. According to the postulates, a link
between agent and disease is valid when (1) the organism is regularly found in
the lesions of the disease, (2) the organism can be isolated in pure culture on
artificial media, (3) inoculation of this culture produces a similar disease in
experimental animals, and 4) the organism can be recovered from the lesions
in these animals. These postulates require modification for viruses, however,
because they cannot be grown on artificial media (viruses require living cells

for their replication) and some are pathogenic only for humans. Nevertheless, these experiments with ferrets, humans, and influenza filled the bill for a modified Koch's postulate. Interestingly, the ferrets originally reported sick in the Wellcome laboratories were subsequently shown to have had canine distemper, not influenza. Considering the role serendipity played in the use of ferrets and the initial isolation of human influenza virus, one agrees with Pasteur: "Chance favors the prepared mind."

Macfarlane Burnet, the eminent Australian scientist, whose contributions to poliomyelitis virus research were mentioned in Chapter 7, was to play an important role in the investigation of influenza. From 1933, when human influenza was isolated, until the early to mid-1950s, when tissue culture systems became available, Burnet pioneered both the technology and conceptual approaches to using embryonated eggs for the study of influenza (22–24) and other viruses. This model became the standard for investigating viral replication and genetic manipulations. Hemagglutination, that is, the clumping of red blood cells, is a simple and reliable test for establishing the presence of many viruses. The principle of hemagglutination was first uncovered when George Hirst of the New York Public Health Institute accidentally tore the blood vessel of an influenza-infected chicken (25,26). Red blood cells escaping from the wound agglutinated, or clumped, around influenza viruses in the infected fluid. From this simple event, Hirst realized that hemagglutination could signal the presence of virus.

The influenza viruses that afflict humans are divided into three types: A, B, and C. Influenza A is responsible for the epidemics and infects not only man but also pigs, horses, seals, and a large variety of birds (3,6). Indeed, influenza A has been isolated worldwide from both domestic and wild birds, primarily waterbirds including ducks, geese, terns, and gulls and domesticated birds such as turkeys, chickens, quail, pheasants, geese, and ducks. Studies of wild ducks in Canada from 1975 to 1994 indicated that up to 20 percent of the juveniles were infected, and fecal samples from their lakeshore habitats contained the virus. These birds usually shed the virus from five to seven days (with a maximum of thirty days) after becoming infected even though they show no sign of the disease. Obviously, this virus and its hosts have adapted mutually over many centuries and created a reservoir that ensures perpetuation of the virus. Duck virus has been implicated in outbreaks of influenza in animals such as seals, whales, pigs, horses, and turkeys. Extensive analysis of the virus's genetic structure, or nucleic acid sequences, supports the hypotheses that mammalian influenza viruses, including those infecting man, may well originate in aquatic birds.

Influenza A viruses from aquatic birds grow poorly in human cells, and vice versa. However, both avian and human influenza viruses can replicate in pigs. We have known that pigs are susceptible to influenza viruses that infect man ever since the veterinarian J. S. Koen first observed pigs with influenza symptoms closely resembling those of humans. Retrospective tests of human blood indicate that the swine virus isolated by Shope in 1928 was similar to the human virus and likely responsible for the human epidemic. Swine influenza still persists year-round and is the cause of most respiratory diseases in pigs. Interestingly, in 1976, swine influenza virus isolated from military recruits at Fort Dix was indistinguishable from virus isolates obtained from a man and a pig on a farm in Wisconsin. The examiners concluded that animals, especially aquatic birds and pigs, can be reservoirs of influenza virus. When such viruses or their components mix with human influenza virus, dramatic genetic shifts can follow, creating the potential of a new epidemic for humans.

The influenza virus continually evolves by antigenic shift and drift. Early studies in this area by Robert Webster and Graeme Laver established the importance of monitoring influenza strains in order to predict future epidemics (27–29). Antigenic shifts are major changes in the structure of the influenza virus that determines its effect on immune responses. Of the viral proteins, the hemagglutinin (H), a major glycoprotein of the virus, plays a central role in infection, because, as mentioned at the beginning of this chapter, breakdown of hemagglutinin into two smaller units is required for virus infectivity. Shifts in the composition of the hemagglutinin (H) or neuraminidase (N), another glycoprotein, of influenza virus were observed in the 1933, 1957, 1968, and 1977 epidemics:

1933: H1N1
1957: H2N2 (Asian flu)
1968: H3N2 (Hong Kong flu)
1977: reappearance of H1N1, called the Russian flu

The reappearance in 1977 of the Russian flu, a virus first isolated in 1933, raises the uneasy possibility that a return of the 1918–19 influenza epidemic with its devastation of human life is possible and perhaps likely.

In March of 1997, part of influenza virus nucleic acid was isolated from a formalin-fixed lung tissue sample of a twenty-one-year-old Army private that died during the 1918–19 Spanish influenza pandemic (30). Since the first influenza viruses were not isolated until the 1930s, characterization of the 1918–19 strain relied on molecular definition of the virus's RNA. Chemical evidence indicated a novel H1N1 sequence of a viral strain that differed from all other subsequently characterized influenza strains and that the 1918 HA

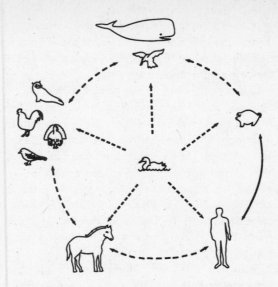

Figure 14.5 The reservoir of influenza A viruses. Wild aquatic birds are believed to be the primary reservoir for avian and mammalian species. Solid lines indicate the known transmission to man from pigs; dashes show possible spread. Diagram courtesy of Rob Webster.

human sequence correlated best with swine influenza strains. Once the entire sequence is on hand, a virulent marker for the influenza virus associated with killing over 675,000 Americans from 1918 to 1919 may be uncovered and a vaccine planned that might abort the return of this virus form of influenza.

When such antigenic shifts occur, the appearance of disease is predictable. Therefore, surveillance centers have been established all over the world where isolates of influenza are obtained and studied for alterations, primarily in the hemagglutinin. According to the evidence from these centers, isolates identified in late spring are excellent indicators of potential epidemics in the following winter.

Both avian and human influenza viruses can replicate in pigs, and genetic reassortants or combinations between them can be demonstrated experimentally. A likely scenario for such an antigenic shift in nature occurs when the prevailing human strain of influenza A virus and an avian influenza virus concurrently infect a pig, which serves as a mixing vessel. Reassortants containing genes derived mainly from the human virus but with a hemagglutinin and polymerase gene from the avian source are able to infect humans and initiate a new pandemic. In rural southeast Asia, the most densely populated area of the world, hundreds of millions of people live and work in close contact with domesticated pigs and ducks. This is the likely reason for influenza pandemics in China. Epidemics other than the 1918–19 catastrophe have generally killed 50,000 or fewer individuals, although within a year over one million people had been infected with these new strains.

Three major hypotheses have been put forth to explain antigenic shifts. First, as described above, a new virus can come from a reassortant in which an avian influenza virus gene substitutes for one of the human influenza virus genes. The genome of human influenza group A contains eight RNA segments, and current wisdom is that the circulating influenza hemagglutinin in humans has been replaced with an avian hemagglutinin. A second explanation for antigenic shifts that yield new epidemic viruses is that strains from other mammals or birds become infectious for humans. Some believe that this is the cause of the Spanish influenza virus epidemic in 1918–19, with the transmission of swine influenza virus to humans. A third possibility is that newly emerging viruses have actually remained hidden and unchanged somewhere but suddenly come forth to cause an epidemic, as the Russian H1N1 virus once did. H1N1 first was isolated in 1933, then disappeared when replaced by the Asian H2N2 in 1957. However, twenty years later the virus reappeared in a strain isolated in northern China and subsequently spread to the rest of the world. This virus was identical in all its genes to one that caused human influenza epidemics in the 1950s. Where the virus was for twenty years is not known. Could it have been inactivated in a frozen state, preserved in an animal reservoir, or obscured in some other way? If this is so, will the Spanish influenza virus also return, and what will be the consequences for the human population?

In addition to antigenic shift, which signifies major changes in existing viruses, antigenic drift permits slight alterations in viral structure. These follow pinpoint changes (mutations) in amino acids in various antigen domains that relate to immune pressure, leading to selection. For example, the hemagglutinin molecule gradually changes while undergoing antigenic drift. Such mutations allow the virus to escape from attack by antibodies generated during a previous bout of infection. Because these antibodies would ordinarily protect the host by removing the virus, this escape permits the related infection to remain in the population.

With these difficulties of antigenic shift and, drift and animal reservoirs, it is not surprising that making an influenza vaccine as effective as those for smallpox, poliovirus, yellow fever, or measles is difficult to achieve. Another complication is that immunity to influenza virus is incomplete; that is, even in the presence of an immune response, influenza can still occur. Nevertheless, the challenge of developing vaccines based on surveillance studies has been met. A chemically treated, formalin-inactivated virus has been formulated in a vaccine that is 30 to 70 percent effective in increasing resistance to influenza virus. The vaccine decreases the frequency of influenza attacks or, at least, the severity of disease in most recipients, although protection is not absolute. In addition, the secondary bacterial infections that may accompany influenza are today treatable with potent antibacterial drugs previously unavailable. Nonetheless, of the plagues that visit humans, influenza is among those that require constant surveillance, because we can be certain that some form of influenza will continue to return.

CHAPTER 15

CONCLUSIONS AND
FUTURE PREDICTIONS

From the mid-nineteenth to early twentieth century, the understanding that microbes, not miasmas or ill winds, caused infectious diseases of humans led to euphoric prophecies that man now had the power to vanquish plagues from our midst. Yet in 1926, when Paul deKruif's classical book *Microbe Hunters* (1) was published, almost every viral disease continued unabatedly and relentlessly to claim victims. An effective vaccine against smallpox had been available since the early 1800s, yet millions of people continued to die from that infection each year, including the year deKruif's book was published. Even though attenuated vaccines could protect chickens from fowl cholera or humans from rabies, medical doctors had no vaccine to use against measles, yellow fever, or poliomyelitis, and these infections continued to kill or cripple. It was true that understanding the biological cycle of yellow fever infection led to public health measures to reduce or eliminate the mosquito vector and that by the early twentieth century control of this infection had increased dramatically. Yet Paul deKruif remained pessimistic, even resigning his research position at the Rockefeller Institute in the early 1920s. In his autobiography, *The Sweeping Wind*, published in 1962, he wrote:

> What was the use of knocking myself out at microbe hunting these days of the beginning 1920s when the universal life-saving advances predicted by the immortal Pasteur seem to have come to a dead end? . . . The blooming golden days of the old microbe hunters were done.
>
> What had become of the brave prophecy of Pasteur's—that it was now in the power of men to make microbic maladies vanish from the face of the globe? . . . Where were the hopes for preventive vaccines? (2)

But deKruif spoke too soon, because fifty to sixty years later, smallpox, yellow fever, measles, and poliomyelitis were under control as he could never have visualized.

Edward Jenner too would have been discouraged had he known how long the wait would be between his great discovery of a vaccine against smallpox and eradication of the disease. In 1800, only four years after his success, he wrote:

> May I not with perfect confidence congratulate my country and society at large on the beholding—an antidote that is capable of extirpating from the earth a disease which is every hour devouring its victims; a disease that has ever been considered as the severest scourge of the human race!

Some 177 years passed before the world's last case of endemic smallpox occurred in Somalia, although in the next year a laboratory accident in Birmingham, England, led to the death of one person. Nevertheless, by 1979, a global commission formed to evaluate the control of smallpox certified that smallpox had been conquered. The Thirty-third World Health Assembly in 1980 accepted this final report and the certification of smallpox eradication. Thus came fulfillment of the first part of Pasteur's prophecy.

With the total elimination of smallpox infection in nature, the debate shifts to a new focus. Should smallpox as a species be removed from our planet? Opinions on this matter are mixed, and in 1999 a special World Health Organization (WHO) committee will meet again to decide this issue. Several arguments against destruction of smallpox stocks remain on the table. First, although depositories in the United States and in Russia continue to sequester stocks of this virus for research, who can ensure that rogue states or societies have not secretly stockpiled the infectious agent elsewhere? Even the elimination of smallpox from these two sites may not keep the agent from reappearing. Although there are now better biological warfare agents than smallpox, it may be quixotic to think that others with secret caches will abandon their supply. This possibility suggests the second issue, the risk of a continuously expanding human population that is susceptible to smallpox. A third argument is that the functions of most of the genes of smallpox are not known. The majority of these genes are not concerned with the virus's basic replication strategy per se, but rather function to alter the infected host so as to favor the virus. These products may prove to have therapeutic value in humans with other diseases. Last, there is the intellectual concern that all living things are part of the cosmic universe and to regard any form of life as a foe and eliminate it from the universe will one day be considered poor philosophy for all. However, unless postponed or altered, many believe that the consensus decision by the WHO Board of Experts will be to eradicate all stocks of smallpox viruses.

This debate does not end with smallpox but will soon encompass poliomyelitis and measles viruses. Both viruses have been targeted for elimination in the early twenty-first century by WHO and the scientific community.

Eradication of infections caused by poliovirus seems feasible within the projected timetable. In 1994 almost 80 percent of children under one year of age throughout the world were immunized against poliomyelitis through the Expanded Program of Immunization (EPI) (3). During 1995 half the world's children under five, roughly 300 million, were immunized as part of the plan to eradicate the disease globally before the year 2005 and possibly as early as 2000. As part of this grand campaign, and reflecting what can be done with active collaboration and goodwill among countries, WHO, other health organizations, medical doctors, and pharmaceutical houses immunized over 160 million children in India and China during just two weeks of December 1995. A month earlier, in war-torn Sri Lanka and in Afganistan in 1996, a short truce was arranged. Called a day of tranquillity, it was organized to enable children on both sides of the conflict to be immunized. The model for this and other programs is the successful campaign that eradicated smallpox in 1979. To accomplish that goal, widespread immunization programs were enforced. In addition, when a case of smallpox was uncovered, everyone around the infected individual was vaccinated. But poliovirus infection differs from smallpox in an important way. The symptoms of smallpox are easily recognized, yet fewer than one in 100 persons infected with poliovirus shows any manifestation of the disease. For that reason, a poliovirus eradication campaign will require near-universal immunization. Nevertheless, it is likely that the poliomyelitis virus will be the second infection totally eliminated from mankind. This will be a great event in human history and should be honored as such. Indeed, in 1997 the WHO Steering Committee involved in vaccination and eradication of polio and measles virus infections heard that in 1996 only 2,090 cases of poliomyelitis occurred worldwide.

With measles virus infection, eradication may be more difficult; it is scheduled for the year 2013. Although the current vaccine is excellent, several scientific advisors to WHO are not confident that it will be effective enough for total elimination of the virus. I am among those advisors who share this concern. But why this divergence of opinion? Measles remains one of the major childhood killers, accounting for more child deaths than all other vaccine-preventable diseases combined (3). Yet of all the vaccines currently administered by EPI and WHO, measles virus when compared with the other five vaccines for childhood diseases administered has the lowest degree of protection (3). Why is the measles virus vaccine so much less effective?

All agree that the current measles virus vaccine has a proven track record of success, strongly arguing in favor of its ability to eradicate measles virus infection. For example, before the EPI launched its vaccination campaign in 1974, the death rate from measles virus was eight million individuals per year. By 1990 global immunization reached 80 percent coverage, and the associated mortality dropped nearly eightfold. Death rates for the last several years are at a low of slightly more than one million individuals per year. Even better, parts of the Caribbean and Central and South America have had virtually no new cases of measles. In 1996, the Pan-American Organization and Centers for Disease Control observed the total eradication of measles virus in Cuba following enforceable national vaccine days. Nevertheless, as long as 200,000 or fewer susceptible persons are available in any one place—the number believed required for the continued circulation of measles virus in an area—there will always be a risk of reinfection. Vaccine coverage is still incomplete not only in Third World countries but also in some industrial countries. For example, in 1994, in some regions of Japan and France coverage of susceptible inhabitants was less than 70 and 60 percent, respectively, and in Italy there was only approximately 50 percent vaccine coverage.

Even so, what is the problem with the current attenuated vaccine? Unlike the poliomyelitis vaccine, which is effective within the first few months of life, the attenuated measles vaccine is not effective early in life. Babies carry antibodies to measles virus from their mothers, and these antibodies inactivate the vaccine for the first six to nine months of life. Therefore, even if the current vaccine is doing most of the job, work to produce a better vaccine that will not be inactivated by antibodies from the mother should continue so that an alternative is available. Further, measles virus suppresses the host's immune response.

When *Microbe Hunters* was published in 1926, no one knew that viruses caused influenza or that infections by the hemorrhagic viruses and HIV lay in the future. Today, monitoring stations worldwide watch for newly emerging variants of the influenza virus and for the return of well-known types. The recent appearance of the hemorrhagic fever viruses and HIV provide current challenges to a new generation of microbe hunters, as did smallpox, poliomyelitis, measles virus, and yellow fever to medical researchers in the past. Evolving viruses, whose mutations cause changes in their genomes, combined with the intrusion of human populations in new agricultural and forest lands, generate new infectious agents and new infectious diseases. With the appropriate resources to do the work, talent to undertake the task, and continuing technologic advances, the viruses causing hemorrhagic fevers should be as controllable as smallpox, yellow fever, measles, and poliomyelitis viruses. However, HIV or other similar infections provide unique problems and stand apart from what has been observed earlier. HIV infection continues in the presence of an anti-HIV immune response. It is likely that the approaches developed that have successfully tamed acute viral infections (smallpox, yellow fever, measles, and poliomyelitis) will have to be modified and rethought to control persistent viral infections.

Since 1953, when James Watson and Francis Crick discovered the structure of DNA, the molecule that contains genetic directions and transmits them from one generation to the next, scientific dogma has asserted that all genetic information is encoded by nucleic acids. However, the recent revelation of prion proteins introduced a new player into microbiology: Some argue that this protein can also provide genetic directions from one generation to the next. Once dismissed as impossible and heretical, the theory that prion forms can transmit disease has gained ever wider acceptance and scientific converts. Prions arise as a result of mutations in a normal cell gene, and some believe that the conformational change from a normal prion to an abnormal one is the cause of spongiform encephalopathies. The prion, in itself, could be the infectious agent able to transmit disease. Current interest focuses on the possibility that prion disease of cows, the bovine spongiform encephalopathy, or mad cow disease, can cross the species barrier and affect humans, leading to progressive dementia and death. A related suggestion is that prions are the cause of other diseases of aging. At issue is not the "scare" value of this information but the prospect of scientific inquiry that will eventually identify and overcome the disease agent.

Using a different strategy, certain viruses infect cells without killing them and, instead, cause a persistent infection. During this long-lived infection viruses can alter the cells' functions. For example, viruses can prevent nerve cells from making molecules necessary for cognitive function and behavior, inhibit endocrine cells from making hormones needed to maintain normal metabolism and growth, and block the immune system from making cytokines, other growth factors, and antibodies required for maintaining protection against microbes and cancers. Research is currently focused on the molecular basis of how these afflictions occur and whether similar diseases affecting the brain, endocrine and immune system, heart and other organs occur in humans.

In the final analysis, the history of viruses, plagues, and people is the history of our world and the events that shaped it. It is also a history of individuals who worked toward the conquest of viruses and the diseases they cause. From the time of Pasteur's great discovery of living vaccines, a large cadre of men and women have joined in the battle against viruses. Their great legacy to our society is that diseases that once took millions of lives with ease have now been controlled or eradicated. In the end, the splendor of human history is not in wars won, dynasties formed or financial empires built, but in the improvement of the human condition. The obliteration of diseases that impinge on our health is a regal yardstick of civilization's success, and those who accomplish that task will be among the true navigators of a brave new world.

AFTERNOTES

PERSPECTIVE

As viruses evolve and new types emerge, so our perceptions continuously change about their potential for hatching plagues. What can and should be done? Since publication of this book in 1998, we now have to face the possible return of smallpox and its use as a weapon of bio-terrorism (1). We have witnessed the return of yellow fever to the United States, the first case in seventy-four years. The vector that spreads that disease, the *Aedes aegypti* mosquito, now dwells in our midst. Even as the march to eradicate poliomyelitis from our world continues at an impressive pace, containment of measles has encountered bumps and setbacks along the way. Measles viruses now infect humans in the tens of thousands in Brazil and in the hundreds of thousands in Japan. The return of measles epidemics highlights its near universal infectivity (>99%) for susceptible populations, the growing pool of susceptible individuals, and the difficulty in eliminating the virus. Since immunization, paralytic poliomyelitis has disappeared from the Americas. Correspondingly, since 1991, the world's total number of recorded cases has diminished more than 89 percent, from over 35,000 to about 2,000 currently. More than two-thirds of children under five years of age, approximately 420 million individuals worldwide, have been vaccinated over the last two years. The hope is that by the year 2002, or by 2005, sufficient immunizations will have blanketed the globe's population to wipe out the poliomyelitis virus.

Yet even now immunization must be required and occur not only in Third World countries but also in the United States. As an example, when Dirk Kempthorne, current governor of Idaho, decided to enhance vaccination of susceptible children, he appointed Jim Hawkins to oversee the program. Because Hawkins was infected with the poliomyelitis virus as a child, he knows its horrors well. Despite this, he is confronted with opposition groups from the Christian Coalition, some other religious factions, and antigovernment groups who do not want any agency or government telling them what to do with their children. As a consequence, the pool of unvaccinated children grows, and the risk to all citizens increases. Currently, Idaho ranks low among states, with only 70 percent coverage for its children. This danger prevails despite proof that protection through immunization succeeds only when the numbers of susceptible people decrease.

Recently in Malaysia, an outbreak of disease from a "mysterious virus" killed over 100 people. The CDC recently identified the virus as a member of the paramyxovirus family to which measles belongs. Further defined as a Hendravirus, this agent resembles the one that attacked two individuals in Queensland, Australia, as described in Chapter 9. The Australian Hendravirus is associated with horses and spread by bats, while the Malaysian Hendra-like virus is associated with pigs.

These newfound viruses, so far, afflict relatively few persons in limited areas of the world, but the human immunodeficiency virus (HIV) continues its devastating march; AIDS, the disease HIV causes, has already killed 10 to 25 percent of the population in regions of Africa and is reported with increasing regularity in Asia. In Western countries, although no individual is yet considered cured of AIDS, aggressive antiviral triple-drug therapy has dramatically reduced the expected death rate. Even so, persisting HIV infection endures in these patients' bodies. Also on the rise is the human form of "mad cow" disease, as prion disease, a variant of Creutzfeldt-Jakob disease, is called. Several new cases appeared in the United Kingdom and one in France last year. This stepwise increase suggests to epidemiologists that rather than a few sporadic cases, a widespread epidemic is now more of a distinct possibility. Because of the long term incubation period for prion disease, it is too early to answer that question now, but it will be answered if cases continue to increase over the next few years (2). An advisory board in the United States concerned with monitoring the safety of the country's blood supply is considering banning persons who lived in England during the mad cow disease epidemic from donating blood to blood banks. The suspicion is, though not yet proven, that blood may retain this agent, which could then be passed via transfusions.

Lastly, fear of a new influenza plague occurred in late 1998, when a novel influenza virus, which killed a third of those it infected, was found to contain an outer glycoprotein coat protein—the hemagglutinin—of birds. This influenza virus protein had never before been isolated in humans (3,4). Fortunately, this time around, the virus that jumped from birds to humans failed to spread from human to human. Further, the major source of this human disease was pinpointed to poultry markets in Hong Kong. The rapid elimination of more than one million ducks, geese, and chickens removed a large reservoir of the virus, thereby preventing the infection of more humans and the eventual evolution of a variant that could spread among human populations, as occurred in the massive influenza epidemic of 1918–1919. With this background, the search intensified to find and identify the 1918–1919 flu virus to learn what made it so deadly. Just below the Arctic Circle and in Alaska, scientists made energetic attempts to obtain permanently frozen tissues from victims of the 1918–1919 outbreak in anticipation that their corpses would contain nucleic acid fingerprints from the virus (5). If the RNA was not degraded, current technology could isolate the viral sequence and the secret of its lethal effects might be decoded. This information would provide the framework for designing countermeasures to minimize its effect if and when the virus reappeared, as discussed in more depth below. However, knowledge of the sequence of the killer influenza still might not by itself shed the light needed to understand the biology or how the virus worked within the infected person.

SMALLPOX

As stated at the end of Chapter 4, the eradication of smallpox depends on the political and economic wherewithal and human desire to do so. Scientific research has provided the tools.

But could eradication fail? Could smallpox return? The virus's natural host is man. There are no animal intermediates, and, since the virus does not linger in the form of a persistent infection, it is amenable to permanent eradication—that is to say, removal from the world. But because the virus no longer circulates in any community, the numbers of never vaccinated or infected susceptible individuals increases. Further, complete or efficient immunity of those previously vaccinated is believed to wane in ten to twenty years. Consequently, the pool of highly susceptible individuals enormously expands.

In the last few years, some countries and individuals have actually chosen to develop more dangerous smallpox viruses by inserting materials alongside its genes. For example, the Soviet Biologic-Weapons Program near Novasbirsk in Western Siberia continued such work using a component of Ebola virus, despite attempts from Gorbachev to curtail it. With the breakup of the Soviet Union, government-funded research decreased dramatically, and scientists working in biowarfare programs often found themselves without jobs. Some went abroad looking for employment by the highest bidder. Several emigrated to the United States or Great Britain as consultants in the defense against such biological weapons, even as the Offensive Biological Weapons Program was discontinued in the United States during the Nixon presidency. Others, perhaps mercenary biologists, have simply disappeared from Russia. One can only guess that they ended up in Iraq, Syria, Libya, Iran, or perhaps other areas with their stocks of smallpox and their technical knowledge to initiate and expand a bioweapons program. However, no one really knows where they are. But because of that threat, several specialists who earlier led the fight to remove smallpox from our planet and destroy the virus as a species have recently advised that funds be earmarked to stockpile vaccines against smallpox and other pathogens and to keep the deadly virus in the United States and Russian designated laboratories. The Clinton administration agreed in late 1998 to request $300 million for this purpose. Implicit in the goal of eradication and elimination of smallpox or other plaque-inducing agents is the need not to vaccinate the population. The billions of dollars saved by not having to make or use vaccines would then be available to control other health problems. Also advised is the retraining of physicians and public health officials in diagnosis of smallpox.

The last natural case of smallpox occurred in 1977 in Somalia at a time when many countries had already discontinued routine vaccination. All countries ceased vaccination programs eight years later in. However, in 1978, a photographer working at the University of Birmingham, England, became infected and died. Supposedly, the source of infection was a secure laboratory for smallpox research located a considerable distance from the room in which the photographer worked. This lethal episode emphasizes the danger of any viable smallpox virus during the posteradication era. As a result of that accident, all strains of smallpox stored in laboratories were supposedly destroyed or transferred to depositories at CDC in Atlanta or the Research Institute for Viral Preparations in Moscow. The World Health Organization Ad Hoc Committee established to deal with this issue recommended in 1986 and 1994 that all remaining smallpox stocks in Atlanta and Moscow be destroyed if no serious objections were received from the international health community and that vaccination to protect military personnel be terminated. Despite the passage of years, neither recommendation has been implemented, and a meeting convened in 1999 to reconsider the issue.

Although humans and their collective institutions have the power to do dramatic good, some have the ability to do overwhelming evil. For the latter reason, smallpox, one of the most intently studied viruses in the past and the killer of millions, could reappear. In recent years, smallpox disease has become more of a curiosity than a medical issue and has been removed from teaching curriculums of some medical schools. Nevertheless, the possibility remains that smallpox in the hands of evildoers will resurface to be seen once again by practitioners of medicine.

YELLOW FEVER

Yellow fever has returned to the United States after an absence of seventy-two years (6). In July 1996, a forty-five-year-old Tennessean vacationed in Brazil, but neglected to receive the mandatory vaccination for yellow fever. During a nine-day fishing trip on the Amazon and Rio Negro rivers, he was bitten by a mosquito carrying the yellow fever virus. Upon return to Knoxville, he developed fever and chills, as Kate Bionda did in Memphis ninety-eight years earlier, when the yellow fever virus also entered her blood, then set off an epidemic (see Chapter 5). Similarly, he deteriorated, vomited blood, and died. As with the Memphis outbreak in 1878, the *Aedes aegypti* mosquito was now loose in Knoxville. But unlike that earlier plague, no other yellow fever infections developed. However, from 1996 to 1997, 254 cases of yellow fever resulted in 103 deaths in South America, including in Brazil, where the virus is endemic, where the mosquito dwells, and where the Tennessee traveler was infected.

NEWLY EMERGING PLAGUES

HEMORRHAGIC FEVER VIRUSES:
EBOLA AND HANTA

Despite careful analysis of thousands of samples from vertebrates, invertebrates, and mammals surrounding the person identified as the index case of the 1995–1996 Ebola virus outbreak in Africa, the source of this virus, how it is transmitted to humans, and exactly how it dissolves tissues are not known. In the Democratic Republic of the Congo (formerly called Zaire), in the city of Kikwit, 30 percent of doctors and 10 percent of nurses caring for patients also developed Ebola hemorrhagic fever, resulting in the Kikwit Hospital's being closed. But perhaps the novel, even defining, event of this local epidemic was the rapid gathering of an international press corp. Live television coverage in Kikwit to countries oceans removed from the Congo created a unique milieu for worldwide information that facilitated a rapid and timely mobilization of experts, equipment, supplies, and even funds for medical investigators. This coverage, the first of its kind, ended a period in history when researchers and physicians surrounded by acute lethal disease worked in relative isolation and obscurity. Instead, the care given these patients and the description of their disease were exposed to detailed scrutiny, often unwarranted. The time scale was as follows. The initial effects of Ebola virus in Kikwik were traced to January 1995. Thirteen weeks later, a district health worker wrote to the national government authorities about a serious outbreak of gastrointestinal disease. The government agency failed to respond, and three weeks later, as the outbreak continued to expand, the government was again notified. Eventually, on 10 May, a World Health Organization (WHO) team of experts arrived. Workers from Medicine Without Frontiers arrived the next day, followed in one more day by medical experts from the CDC and Pasteur Institute. Amazingly, the first journalists and TV crews arrived the following day, or three days after the initial arrival of the WHO team. According to Heymann et al., "[T]hey arrived on small chartered planes, often violating many of the protective barriers against the spread of disease with the purpose to . . . get the most sensational stories or photographs . . . often displaying questionable ethical standards . . . not obtaining permission to film or photograph or ignoring and compounding family grief, family members grieving for the sick, burying the dead . . . often disrupting treatment and care, and often leading to increased costs because of their (press) use of supplies and vehicles. . . ." (7) The days of isolation and age of innocence, taking care of patients and in performing research on plagues, had passed. Health workers realized the need to arrange daily press briefings and nonintrusive access to accurate photographic sessions. In May 1999 more than sixty deaths with a picture similar to Ebola occurred in the Congo. However, this time not Ebola but deadly Marburg virus was the cause, a virus not seen since 1975 in Zimbabwe, where it infected three individuals, resulting in one death (see Chapter 10). It is believed that the current outbreak infected seventy-six people working in mines near the town of Durba in the Congo. Marburg virus obtained its name when a deadly disease occurred in Marburg, Germany, in laboratory personnel working with tissues obtained from African monkeys.

The Reston strain of Ebola virus was responsible for an outbreak of hemorrhagic fever in a facility housing primates outside of Washington, D.C. The virus is believed to have originated in Asia, but exactly where and in what organism are not clear. Reston Ebola is less likely to produce disease in humans and monkeys than the various African Ebola isolates.

The Hantavirus induces a pulmonary disease that is now killing 45 percent of the people infected throughout the United States, but mostly in the Southwest. The belief that this infection spreads only from rodent to man changed during a 1998 outbreak in the El Bolson area of Southern Argentina, when eleven of the twenty people infected by this route died. For the first time, the evidence collected pointed to virus spread from one of these patients to the others. Human-to-human spread in residential areas likely enhances the number of Hantavirus infections, and it presents major difficulties during hospitalization, as isolation of patients is required.

HIV: THE CURRENT PANDEMIC

Less than a year and a half has passed since the original publication of this book, but even in that brief period, several components of HIV infection and AIDS have become uncovered or better defined. The origin of HIV was revealed by a combination of serendipity and exceptional detective work. The inception of HIV-1 was traced to a related virus, simian immunodeficiency virus of chimpanzees (SIVcpz) in a *Pantroglodyte troglodyte* subspecies of chimpanzee (8). As anticipated the natural host, the chimpanzee, lives in equilibrium with the virus and usually does not become ill. SIVcpz jumped to humans likely through chimpanzee bites and/or exposure to virus-contaminated blood during hunting or preparation of food. Beginning in a sparse rural area, it migrated into villages and cities, then spread across continents. HIV now infects over thirty million people in the world. From this observation, at least three fundamental questions arise. First, do the different outcomes of infection in humans (illness leading to progressive disease [AIDS] and death) and in chimpanzees (no disease) result from tiny changes in the genetic make-up of the virus or of the host? Second, why or how does the chimpanzee's immune system resist the damning effects of the virus while, in contrast, the immune system of man is susceptible? Third, could other, similar animal viruses in nature cause future diseases and plagues for humans; if so, can we find such agents and disarm them before they infect humans?

The pivotal detective work on HIV-1 came from the study of a chimpanzee named Marilyn that died in 1985 but had been infected with SIVcpz for over twenty-six years without progressing to AIDS. In 1959, Marilyn, captured in Africa, was transported to the United States to serve in a breeding program of chimpanzees to be used for research projects. Shortly after the discovery of HIV in 1985, some chimpanzees to be used for developing and evaluating an AIDS vaccine were first bled for baseline values. Their blood was then screened to determine if they had been infected (had evidence of antibodies) with HIV. Of the chimpanzees screened, only Marilyn was found to be infected, but she died shortly thereafter. Samples of her tissue were sent to the National Cancer Institute (NCI) of the National Institutes of Health (NIH) for study. However, no virus was recovered from these tissues, and the autopsy showed no evidence of HIV-related disease. The remaining tissue was then frozen. Ten years later, in 1995, entirely by serendipity, a scientist trying to obtain additional freezer space for his own work began to inspect and discard old stored tissues. He noted Marilyn's tissues, knew of Dr. Beatrice Hahn's (University of Alabama, Birmingham) interest in searching for the origin of HIV-1, and contacted her to see if she was interested in receiving Marilyn's tissues. Hahn knew that this was a unique opportunity because SIVcpz infection had previously been found in only three chimpanzees of the nearly four hundred studied. In fact, one of the SIVcpz species was so different from HIV-1, according to genetic analysis, that a direct link seemed unlikely. Now, in contrast, Hahn's studies showed a close correlation between the SIVcpz isolated from Marilyn and HIV-1. The next step taken revealed that three of the four SIVcpz isolates came from *Pantroglodytes troglodytes* and that these three showed similarities in structure to HIV. Lastly, the natural habitat for *Pantroglodytes troglodytes* was in West and central Africa, the areas where HIV-1 was first identified.

As exciting as news of the likely origin of HIV-1 was, it shared the stage with a scandal involving HIV-infected blood and the alarming increase in AIDS patients. In 1985, three French ministers, Laurent Fabius (former Prime Minister), Georgina Dufoix (former Prime Minister of Society Affairs), and Edmond Herve (former Secretary of State for Health) went on trial for supplying HIV-contaminated blood to the public. They were accused of involuntary homicide for delaying the introduction of a test developed by Robert Gallo in the United States for screening blood, because they wished to protect the market for the development of a competitive French test. During this unsavory period, 4,400 people became infected with HIV, and about 40 percent eventually died. An emotional trial was fueled by the media, families, and victims. For example, Soleine Paugham, a lawyer from the Association of Hemophiliacs, stated on national television, "Involuntary homicide does not satisfy me one bit because I think that nothing was involuntary and everything was on purpose in this affair. . . ." Additional factors were the "lack of serious judicial investigation" and the "visible lack of grasp of the incidence and charge . . . (by the court). . . ." The scientific journal *Nature* called this trial a "French Farce," characterizing the judgment to exonerate as not one of individuals but of the entire system of ruling elites and advisors, usually all graduates from prestigious grandes écoles (9).

The news from Africa is not good. Of over thirty million people worldwide with HIV in 1998, twenty-one million were in Africa. Zimbabwe had the highest incidence, with over 25 percent of its population infected. Botswana had similar incidence of the disease. If HIV killed rapidly, instead of over a ten- to fifteen-year period, it would resemble the influenza plague of 1918–1919 or the Black Death plague of the Middle Ages that reduced the population of Europe by one-fourth. Currently, one-third of adults in several major African cities are infected, nearly 70 percent of whom are females. In many prenatal clinics, the infectivity rate ranges from 30 to 45 percent, and 1.6 million children each year lose at least one parent to AIDS. In East Africa, 40 percent of children fifteen years old or younger have lost mothers or both parents to AIDS.

Reflecting the magnitude of this epidemic is the large number of infected women in their child-bearing years, the large number of children per family, the lack of therapeutic drugs, the sexually permissive society, and the denial of disease. The consequence is near paralysis of Africa's economy. For example, some South African mining companies report 25 percent HIV infection for some shifts. The death rate of Africans employed in Zambia's Barclays Bank is tenfold greater than expected in branches of non-African countries. Similar economic consequences are documented in neighboring Zimbabwe. Most often those infected will die within ten years. In the stronger economies of West Africa (i.e., Nigeria, Ghana, and the Ivory Coast) the incidence of HIV is lower but rising. The result is chaos in health care delivery and public health services. For example, the annual budget for medical care in most African countries is less than $6 per person. Zimbabwe allocates under $4 per individual, but the cost for hospitalization of an insured AIDS patient over the same year is roughly $18,000, and the cost for aggressive triple drug therapy to control HIV replication is close to $15,000. The relatively affluent country of South Africa has difficulty affording the $80 per person required to use the drug AZT for pregnant and nursing mothers to prevent transmission of HIV to their children. In Durban, South Africa, AIDS infects over 40 percent of black children in hospitals, but none are treated with anti-HIV drugs. According to Dr. Hoosen Coovadia, the physician at Durban hospital, his hospital cannot afford the drugs. (Coovadia is to chair the next World AIDS Conference, to be held in Durban.) Often more work hours are lost to attending funerals than for illness. The plight of Africa is dramatically pictured by Michael Specter in a 6 August 1998 *New York Times* article. He describes a funeral in Tshalotsho, Zimbabwe, of an infant who died from AIDS; the child's mother and grandmother attended, but no men. The father had died a few months earlier, his grandfather the previous year, a brother nine years before, and three uncles were also dead—all from AIDS. During the last few years worldwide, six million people have been newly infected, and 2.3 million have died. HIV is now the fifth leading cause of death, and Africa has nearly 90 percent of AIDS-related deaths.

By contrast, in the United States and in Europe, over 100,000 people have been dramatically helped by an aggressive triple drug therapy. The number of people with complications of AIDS has declined, and in the United States the AIDS mortality rate has decreased by almost 50 percent in each of the last two years (10). Yet, no one has been cured, because the virus persists in a dormant state in cells of the immune system.

We in the West, specifically in the United States, have our own house to keep in order. As of 13 March 1999, New York state continued its slow and cautious movement to implement a new HIV reporting and partner notification program. Although every state requires that doctors report AIDS cases to public health officials, not all states report individuals with HIV infection, and most do not require notification of sexual partners by local public health departments or by physicians. Yet medical advances make it imperative for people to know their HIV status, since effective treatments can dramatically slow the progress of AIDS. Even so, partner notifications have been delayed because: 1) no department or person is responsible for the program, 2) neither state or federal government has defined the cost or provided the funds, 3) social ramifications interfere, and 4) some AIDS advocacy groups object to government coertion, limits on individual freedom and threats to job security and insurance coverage. However, a law passed by the New York State Legislature in June 1998 but not yet implemented requires doctors and laboratories to report names and addresses of HIV-positive individuals, as well as names of sexual or needle-sharing partners. An estimated 22,000 HIV-partner notifications are expected annually to the probable 100,000 to 140,000 previously unreported partners. Sadly, the impetus for this law was the case of Nushawn Williams, an HIV-positive man without AIDS, who infected about forty women in New York. Because there was no legal reporting system for HIV-positive non-AIDS persons, no one stopped Williams's activities nor informed those he infected that they may have passed the virus on to other sexual partners. Eventual notification of infected partners and Williams's apprehension occurred only because he also had a venereal disease for which reporting was mandatory. Clearly, this event in recent history confirms that an individual's rights of sexual preference and freedom do not supersede but should go hand-in-hand with society's right to limit the spread of disease.

The contrast in death rates at geographical areas where drug therapy is or is not available for AIDS patients emphasizes that countries lacking resources must receive assistance from the more affluent countries. Rich and poor countries need to provide education on how to prevent the spread of HIV. There is no time left for denial. The epidemic must be recognized everywhere in the world for what it is—a sentencing each day of 16,000 people to a slow and miserable death. Appropriate public health measures and delivery of health care must be supplied.

INFLUENZA:
THE PLAGUE THAT NEARLY RETURNED

On 10 May 1997, a three-year-old child in Hong Kong was admitted to the hospital with influenza virus and died eleven days later. Isolation and characterization of the virus revealed that it was a new human pathogen, formerly known to only infect birds (3,4). By the end of December 1997, eighteen cases were confirmed with a mortality rate of 33 percent. Molecular analysis revealed that the virus's outer coat protein, the influenza hemagglutinin, was of bird origin, typed as hemagglutinin-5. The ability of this avian virus to replicate in humans was surprising and of great concern. Only because this influenza virus failed to adapt sufficiently in humans to allow easy spread from one human to others was a new pandemic stopped. Once the source of this virus was traced to the poultry markets in Hong Kong, over one and a half million domestic birds were quickly slaughtered to prevent possible adaptation of the virus for transmission among humans. By this means the source of the virus was removed, and the potential cycle of adaptation of virus to human was interrupted.

Any new influenza virus capable of replicating in and spreading among humans is a potential candidate for the next influenza pandemic. The only prediction that can be made is that another influenza epidemic is likely to arrive. Continued surveillance of influenza viruses in humans and animals and understanding the mechanism (pathogenesis) that determines host range, host susceptibility, and virulence (strength) of influenza viruses remain the best preparations for preventing and treating the coming plague. Toward that end, new efforts were directed to unlocking the secret of the deadly influenza virus of 1918–1919. The question was, what made that virus so lethal that it killed twenty to forty million people worldwide, including 600,000 within nine months in the United States? This number included one-third of all American physicians. To decipher that mystery, two strategies were used, both made possible through advances in molecular biology. By copying minute amounts of RNA with a molecular technique (reverse transcriptase-polymerase chain reaction), fingerprints of the 1918–1919 influenza virus could be analyzed. The first requirement was tissue from victims of the 1918–1919 epidemic. Accordingly, the lungs from such patients, preserved in fixatives, were used as the source of RNA. This RNA, after extension by a polymerase chain reaction, was subjected to sequencing to identify changes that made the virus so lethal. An alternative second approach was to obtain RNA from tissues of individuals who died during the 1918–1919 plague and were then buried in ice. This would be analogous to the storage of tissues in a freezer. One grave site was found in Brevig Mission, Alaska, where an Inuit Eskimo woman who died in December 1918, was buried in permafrost. At another site, seven hundred miles away from the North Pole in the town of Lonjyearbeen, Norway, were the graves of seven farmers and fishermen, aged eighteen to twenty-nine years, who died of influenza at about the same time. In both the Alaskan and Norwegian locations, during the summer months the top

1 to 1.2 meters of permafrost thaws. If the buried tissue also thawed, the RNA could break down from the action of normal enzymes in the body. Therefore, careful testing of the tissues is essential. Analysis has now begun of RNA from three of those influenza victims, two soldiers whose tissues were preserved at the Armed Forces Institute of Pathology in Washington, and the Inuit woman who was buried in the Alaskan permafrost (5,11). However, because all the influenza genes, including the hemagglutinin, have not yet been completely sequenced, the results of this project are still inconclusive at present. Further, the lethal factor may not reside as expected in the hemagglutinin gene, and the biology of how the virus acted rapidly to kill young adults may not be uncoded from the sequence data.

MAD COW DISEASE: TRANSMISSIBLE SPONGIFORM ENCEPHALOPATHIES

Just fourteen years ago, a new degenerative prion disorder of cattle, bovine spongiform encephalitis (BSE, mad cow disease), was recognized and followed less than four years ago, by discovery of a new variant in humans (Creutzfeldt-Jakob variant [CJV]), a transmissible spongiform encephalitis (TSE) that causes nerve degeneration and death. Since that first documentation of the progressive disease in cattle, more than 170,000 cows in the United Kingdom, several hundred in Switzerland, and lesser numbers in France, the Netherlands, and Portugal were recorded, probably only a fraction of the actual but unreported number. As a consequence, and in an effort to overcome consumer fears about getting mad cow disease (CJV) from eating British beef, over 2.6 million head of cattle were destroyed. Export of British beef was banned, and the British cattle industry suffered near financial ruin. Since lifting of the European Union ban on British beef in 1998, only one-sixth of the preban levels have been exported. The British government still forbids the sale of beef bones, bone marrow, and most cuts of beef on the bone (ribs, T-bone steak). In fact, research proved that BSE can be transmitted orally with an incubation period of two to eight years when cattle are fed TSE-infected meat or bone meal. Concurrently, during the last four years, forty people have died of CJV, thirty-nine in the United Kingdom and one in France, presumably after oral ingestion of the BSE agent (2). The economic outcome is bankruptcy of many farm and livestock businesses, and the political ramifications are that members of the government in power during the outbreak have lost the trust of scientists, the British citizenry, and the European trading partners who purchased and used the contaminated beef. Recent retrospective inquiry by a government panel pointed to gross incompetency by the former Ministry of Agriculture, Fisheries and Food, secrecy and negligence by administrators who knew the danger, and the lack of a scientific advisory board to analyze or publicize the scale of the problem that began in the late 1980s. Even worse, the possibility that BSE might pass to and infect humans was largely ignored (12).

Although proof that CJV originates from BSE is still incomplete, the accumulated evidence indicates that eating diseased beef products was the probable cause. Two separate studies provide reasonable evidence for that conclusion. First, chemical profiles of the prions (abnormally altered proteins) from patients with CJV and/or animals with BSE showed that sugars on the protein were more similar to each other than to prions from other species. Second, when mice were manipulated to produce human prions, the incubation times from introduction of either BSE or CJV prions to onset of disease were similar, as were the location and pattern of disease in the brain; both events differed from those caused by other (non-CJV) human or animal prions. The time required for orally ingested BSE to cause disease in humans is unknown, perhaps ten to twenty years or longer. Therefore, up to twenty years from now a related neurodegenerative disease may increase somewhat, or an epidemic of mad cow disease (CJV) could afflict thousands of humans. Unfortunately, the rapid increase in cases in 1998, compared to 1995 and 1996, does not bode well (2). Another dilemma is whether infectious prions in blood cells or blood products travel to the brain and cause CJV disease. The scientific advisory panel in the United States that evaluates TSE for the Food and Drug Administration, in a split vote, recommended preventing blood donations by anyone exposed to BSE during the epidemic's peak in the United Kingdom. The basis for that recommendation was a research report of prion disease in mice, yet to be confirmed in other laboratories, that TSE could spread through blood. If so, the disaster from HIV-infected blood transfusions could replay for TSE. Although no evidence supports this pathway for transmission of TSE to humans, the panel advised obtaining better epidemiologic data and screening out potential blood donors who may have been exposed to BSE. Estimates are that our nation's blood supply would be reduced approximately 10 percent, requiring replacement of one million donors.

Yet another surprise was in store. In March 1999, a monkey and several lemurs in French zoos grew sick with symptoms reminiscent of mad cow disease (13). Such animals, normally vegetarians, were fed protein supplements containing the rendered remains of British cattle. To evaluate whether these animals could actually develop a prionlike disease associated with BSE, infected cattle brain was fed to two young lemurs that had never before eaten meat; after five months both developed TSE.

With the interest peaking in prion disease and in recognition of its discovery, related scientific work, and identification of human genetic diseases
caused by prions, the Nobel Prize in Physiology and Medicine was awarded
to Stanley Prusiner in December 1997. The award acknowledged the singular purpose and robust contributions Prusiner made in biomedical research
and his discovery of prions—"a new biologic principle of infection." Most
skeptics have been converted to Prusiner's theory stating that passage of
information needed for infection can reside in a protein (14). However, a
nidus of nonconverts continues to view the theory of genetic information
passed by protein instead of nucleic acid as not yet proven (15). These few
contend that the only acceptable proof is conversion of the normal to the
abnormal prion protein in a test tube, followed by using the abnormal protein to cause the disease. How this controversy plays out may only be
resolved in the next millennium.

WORKS CITED

CHAPTER 1: A GENERAL INTRODUCTION

1. D. A. Henderson. "Smallpox Eradication." In *Microbe Hunters Past and Present*, ed. H. Koprowski and M. B. A. Oldstone, pp. 39–43. Bloomington, 1996.
2. Donald Hopkins. *Princes and Peasants: Smallpox in History*. Chicago, 1983.
3. Hugh Thomas. *Conquest: Montezuma, Cortes, and the Fall of Old Mexico*. New York, 1993.
4. William H. McNeill. *Plagues and Peoples*. New York, 1976.
5. Dumas Malone. *Jefferson the President: First Term 1801–1805*. Boston, 1970.
6. J. E. Gibson. *Dr. Bodo Otto and the Medical Background of the American Revolution*. Springfield, 1937.
7. John R. Paul. *A History of Poliomyelitis*. New Haven, 1971.
8. Sven Gard. Presentation speech for the Nobel Award in physiology and medicine, 1954.

CHAPTER 2: INTRODUCTION TO THE PRINCIPLES OF VIROLOGY

1. P. B. Medawar and J. S. Medawar. *Aristotle to Zoos*. Cambridge, 1983.
2. Martin S. Hirsch and James Curran. "Human Immunodeficiency Virus." In *Fields' Virology*, ed. B. N. Fields et al., pp. 1953–76. New York, 1990.
3. Q. J. Sattentau, A. G. Dalgleish, R. A. Weiss, et al. "Epitopes of the CD4 Antigen and HIV Infection." *Science* 234 (1986):1120.
4. Denise Naniche, G. Varior-Krishman, F. Cervoni, et al. "Human Membrane Cofactor Protein (CD46) Acts as a Cellular Receptor for Measles Virus." *J. Virol.* 67 (1993):6025.
5. R. E. Dorig, A. Marcel, A. Chopra, et al. "The Human CD46 Molecule Is a Receptor for Measles Virus (Edmonston Strain)." *Cell* 75 (1993):295.
6. M. Manchester, M. K. Liszewski, J. P. Atkinson, and M. B. A. Oldstone. "Multiple Isoforms of CD46 (Membrane Cofactor Protein) Serve as Receptors for Measles Virus." *Proc. Natl. Acad. Sci. USA* 91 (1994):2161–65.
7. R. Johnstone, B. E. Loveland, and I. F. McKenzie. "Identification and Quantification of Complement Regulator CD46 on Normal Human Tissues." *Immunology* 79 (1993):341.
8. M. B. A. Oldstone. "Virus Neutralization and Virus-Induced Immune Complex Disease: Virus-Antibody Union Resulting in Immunoprotection or Immuno-

logic Injury—Two Sides of the Same Coin." In *Progress in Medical Virology*, Vol. 19, ed. J. L. Melnick, pp. 84–119. Basel, 1975.

9. M. B. A. Oldstone. "Molecular Anatomy of Viral Disease." *Neurology* 37 (1987):453–60.

10. M. B. A. Oldstone. "Viruses and Diseases of the Twenty-first Century." *Amer. J. Pathol.* 143 (1993):1241–49.

11. D. I. Ivanovski. "Ueber die Mosaikkrankheit der Tabakspflanze." *Zentbl. Bakt. ParasitKde*, Abt. II 5 (1899):250–54.

12. M. W. Beijerinck. "Bemerkung zu dem Aufsatz von Herrn Iwanowsky uber die Mosaikkrankheit der Tabakspflanze." *Zentbl. Bakt ParasitKde*, Abt. I 5 (1899):310–11.

13. F. Loeffler and P. Frosch. "Berichte der Kommission zur Erforschung der Maul und Klauenseuche bei dem Institut fur Infektionskrankheiten in Berlin." *Zentbl Bakt ParasitKde*, Abt. I 23 (1898):371–91.

CHAPTER 3: INTRODUCTION TO THE PRINCIPLES OF IMMUNOLOGY

1. J. L. Whitton and M. B. A. Oldstone. "Immune Response to Viruses." In *Fields' Virology*, 3rd ed., ed. B. N. Fields et al., pp. 345–74. Philadelphia, 1996.

2. G. J. V. Nossal. "Life, Death and the Immune System." *Scientific American*, September 1993, pp. 53–62.

3. U. H. Koszinowski, S. Jonjic, and M. J. Reddehase. "The Role of CD4 and CD8 T Cells in Viral Infections." *Curr. Opin. Immunol.* (1991).

4. P. C. Doherty, S. Hou, and R. A. Tripp. "CD8$^+$ T-Cell Memory to Viruses." *Curr. Opin. Immunol.* 6 (1994):545–52.

5. C. A. Biron. "Cytokines in the Generation of Immune Responses to, and Resolution of, Virus Infection." *Curr. Opin. Immunol.* 6 (1994):530–38.

6. M. B. A. Oldstone. "Virus Neutralization and Virus-Induced Immune Complex Disease: Virus-Antibody Union Resulting in Immunoprotection or Immunologic Injury—Two Sides of the Same Coin." In *Progress in Medical Virology*, Vol. 19, ed. J. L. Melnick, pp. 84–119. Basel, 1975.

CHAPTER 4: SMALLPOX

1. F. Fenner and D. A. Henderson. *Smallpox and Its Eradication*. Geneva, 1988.

2. D. A. Henderson. "Smallpox Eradication." In *Microbe Hunters Past and Present*, ed. H. Koprowski and M. B. A. Oldstone, pp. 39–44. Bloomington, 1996.

3. Frank Fenner. "Poxviruses." In *Fields' Virology*, ed. B. N. Fields et al., pp. 2673–702. New York, 1996.

4. William H. McNeil. *Plagues and Peoples*. New York, 1976.

5. Donald Hopkins. *Princes and Peasants: Smallpox in History*. Chicago, 1983.

6. Abbas M. Behbehani. "Life and Death of an Old Disease." *Microb. Rev.* 4 (1983):455.

7. Frank Fenner. "History of Smallpox." In *Microbe Hunters Past and Present*, ed. Koprowski and Oldstone, pp. 25–38.

8. K. C. Wong and L. T. Wu. *History of Chinese Medicine*, 2nd ed. Shanghai, 1936.

9. Rhazes (Al-Razi, Abu Bakr Muhammad). *De Variolis et Morbillis Commentarius*. Londini, G. Bowyer 1766. English translation in *Med. Class.* 4 (1939):22.

10. Hugh Thomas. *Conquest: Montezuma, Cortes, and the Fall of Old Mexico.* New York, 1993.

11. J. Duffy. "Smallpox and the Indians in the American Colonies." *Bull. Hist. Med.* 25 (1951):324.

12. J. A. Poupard and L. A. Miller. "History of Biological Warfare: Catapults to Capsomeres." *Ann. N.Y. Acad. Sci.* 666 (1992):9.

13. H. Bouquet. Letter, June 23, 1763. MSS 21634:295. British Library, London.

14. H. Bouquet. Letter, July 13, 1763. MSS 21634:321. British Library, London.

15. Christopher Ward. *The War of the Revolution.* New York, 1952.

16. H. Thursfield. "Smallpox in the American War of Independence." *Ann. Med. Hist.* 2 (1940):312.

17. J. E. Gibson. *Dr. Bodo Otto and the Medical Background of the American Revolution.* Springfield, 1937.

18. F. Fenner, ed., *The Biology of Animal Viruses.* New York, 1974.

19. Emanuel Timoni. "An Account or History of the Procuring of the Smallpox by Incision or Inoculation: As Has for Some Time Been Practiced at Constantinople." Phil. Trans. Royal Society, 1714.

20. Edward Jenner. *An Inquiry into the Causes and Effects of Variolae Vaccine, a Disease Discovered in Some of the Western Counties of England, Particularly Gloucestershire, and Known by the Name of the Cowpox.* London, 1798.

21. J. B. Blake. *Benjamin Waterhouse and the Introduction of Vaccination.* Philadelphia, 1957.

22. B. Waterhouse. *A Prospect of Exterminating the Smallpox.* Boston, 1800.

23. R. H. Halsey. *How the President, Thomas Jefferson and Dr. Benjamin Waterhouse Established Vaccination as a Public Health Procedure.* History of Medicine Series 5. New York, 1936.

24. Dumas Malone. *Jefferson the President: First Term 1801–1805.* Boston, 1970.

25. Stephen E. Ambrose. *Undaunted Courage,* p. 115. New York, 1996.

26. World Health Organization. Official Records, no. 151. Geneva, Switzerland.

27. Ibid., no. 152.

28. D. A. Henderson. Personal communication, 1995.

CHAPTER 5: YELLOW FEVER

1. J. D. Goodyear. "The Sugar Connection: A New Perspective on the History of Yellow Fever." *Bull. Hist. Med.* 52 (1978).

2. Hugh Thomas. *Conquest: Montezuma, Cortes and the Fall of Old Mexico.* New York, 1993.

3. George K. Strode et al. *Yellow Fever.* New York, 1951.

4. D. S. Freestone. *Yellow Fever Vaccine.* Chapter 27.

5. William H. McNeill. *Plagues and Peoples.* New York, 1976.

6. Henry Rose Carter. *Yellow Fever: An Epidemiological and Historical Study of Its Place of Origin.* Baltimore, 1931.

7. H. Block. "Yellow Fever Epidemic in Philadelphia 1793." *N. Y. State J. Med.* 73 (1973).

8. William Currie. A Description of the Malignant, Infectious Fever Prevailing at Present in Philadelphia; with an Account of the Means to Prevent Infection, and the Remedies and Method of Treatment, Which Have Been Found Most Successful.

9. D. Geggus. "Yellow Fever in the 1790's: The British Army in Occupied Santo Domingo." *Med. Hist.* 23 (1979).

10. John H. Powell. *Bring Out Your Dead. The Great Plague of Yellow Fever in Philadelphia in 1793.* New York, 1970.

11. A. W. Woodruff. *Benjamin Rush, His Work.*

12. Dumas Malone. *Jefferson the President, 1st Term 1801–1805.* Boston, 1970.

13. S. R. Bruesch. "Yellow Fever in Tennessee in 1878." *J. Tenn. Med. Assoc.* 71 (1978); 72 (1979).

14. T. H. Baker. "Yellow Jack: The Yellow Fever Epidemic of 1878 in Memphis, Tennessee." *Bull. Hist. Med.* 42 (1968).

15. J. M. Keating. *A History of the Yellow Fever. The Yellow Fever Epidemic of 1878 in Memphis, Tennessee.* The Howard Association, 1879. Keating was the editor of the newspaper *The Daily Appeal*, as well as an active member in the Howard Association and Citizen's Committee.

16. G. Rosen. *A History of Public Health.* New York, 1958.

17. *The Daily Appeal*, August 13, 1878.

18. *The Sisters of St. Mary at Memphis: With the Acts and Suffering of the Priests and Others Who Were There with Them During the Yellow Fever Season of 1878.* New York, 1879.

19. M. Wingfield. *The Life and Letters of Dr. William J. Armstrong.* West Tennessee Historical Society Papers, Vol. IV, 1956.

20. *The Centennial History of the Tennessee State Medical Association 1830–1930.* Tennessee State Medical Association, 1930.

21. W. Reed and J. Carroll. "The Etiology of Yellow Fever." *Amer. Med.* 3 (1902).

22. A. Agramonte. "The Inside History of a Great Medical Discovery." *Sci. Monthly* 1 (1915).

23. J. Carroll. "Yellow Fever—A Popular Lecture." *Amer. Med.* 9 (1905).

24. J. Carroll. "A Brief Review of the Aetiology of Yellow Fever." *N. Y. Med. J. & Phila. Med. J.* 79 (1904).

25. A. Agramonte. "The Transmission of Yellow Fever." *J. Am. Med. Assoc.* 40 (1903).

26. C. Finlay. "El mosquito hipoteticamenti considerado como agente de transmision

de la fiebre amarella." *Anales de la Real Academia Ciencias Medicas, Fisicas y Naturales de la Habana* 18 (1881).

27. C. Finlay. *Carlos Finlay and Yellow Fever.* New York, 1940.

28. F. Delaporte. *The History of Yellow Fever.* Cambridge, 1991.

29. F. de Lesseps. *Recollections of Forty Years.* New York, 1888.

30. J. C. Rodrigues. *The Panama Canal. Its History, Its Political Aspects and Financial Difficulties.* New York, 1885.

31. I. E. Bennett. *History of the Panama Canal. Its Construction and Builders.* Washington, 1915.

32. D. McCullough. *The Path Between the Seas.* New York, 1977.

33. T. Roosevelt. *An Autobiography.* New York, 1920.

34. A. Stokes, J. Bauer, and N. Hudson. "Experimental Transmission of Yellow Fever to Laboratory Animals." *Am. J. Trop. Med.* 8 (1928).

35. W. Lloyd, M. Theiler, and N. Ricci. "Modification of the Virulence of Yellow Fever Virus by Cultivation in Tissues in Vitro." *Trans. R. Soc. Trop. Med. Hyg.* 29 (1936).

36. W. Sawyer, S. Kitchen, and W. Lloyd. "Vaccination Against Yellow Fever with Immune Serum and Virus Fixed for Mice." *J. Exp. Med.* 55 (1932).

37. M. Theiler and H. Smith. "The Effect of Prolonged Cultivation in Vitro upon the Pathogenicity of Yellow Fever Virus." *J. Exp. Med.* 65 (1937).

38. M. Theiler and H. Smith. "The Use of Yellow Fever Virus Modified by in Vitro Cultivation for Human Immunization." *J. Exp. Med.* 65 (1937).

39. M. Theiler. Nobel Prize in Physiology of Medicine Lecture, 1951.

CHAPTER 6: MEASLES VIRUS

1. William Squire. "On Measles in Fiji." *Trans. Epidem. Soc. (London)* 4 (1877):72.

2. P. Christensen, S. Henning, H. Bang et al. "An Epidemic of Measles in Southern Greenland, 1951. Measles in Virgin Soil." *Acta. Med. Scand.* 144 (1952):430.

3. Erling Norrby and Michael N. Oxman. "Measles Virus." In *Fields' Virology*, ed. B. N. Fields et al., pp. 1013–44. New York, 1990.

4. Laurie E. Markowitz and Samuel L. Katz. "Measles Vaccine." In *Vaccines*, ed. S. A. Plotkin and E. A Mortimer, Jr., pp. 229–76. Philadelphia, 1988.

5. Michael McChesney and Michael B.A. Oldstone. "Virus Induced Immunosuppression: Infections with Measles Virus and Human Immunodeficiency Virus." *Adv. Immunol.* 45 (1989):335.

6. William Osler. *The Principles and Practice of Medicine.* New York, 1904.

7. Clements von Pirquet. "Das Verhalten del kutanen Tuberkulin-Reaktion Wahrend der Masern." *Dtsch. Med. Wochenschr.* 34 (1908):1297.

8. Richard Wagner. *Clements von Pirquet: His Life and Work.* Baltimore, 1968.

9. R. W. Blumberg and H. A. Cassady. "Effect of Measles on Nephrotic Syndrome." *Am. J. Dis. Child.* 63 (1947):151.

10. William H. McNeill. *Plagues and Peoples*. New York, 1976.

11. Hugh Thomas. *Conquest: Montezuma, Cortes and the Fall of Old Mexico*. New York, 1993.

12. Leslie Spie. *Yuma Tribes of the Gila River*. New York, 1970.

13. George Rosen. *A History of Public Health*. New York, 1958.

14. Saul Krugman, J. Giles, A. Jacobs, et al. Studies with the Live Attenuated Measles-Virus Vaccine. *Am. J. Child.* 103 (1962):353.

15. P. L. Panum. *Observations Made During the Epidemic of Measles on the Faeroes Islands in the Year 1846*. New York, 1940.

16. Paul E. Steiner. *Disease in the Civil War*. Springfield, Ill., 1968.

17. H. H. Cuningham. *Doctors in Gray*. Baton Rouge, 1958.

18. The United States Surgeon-General's Office. *The Medical and Surgical History of the War of the Rebellion 1861–1865*. Washington, D.C., 1870–88.

19. Robert E. Lee. *The War of the Rebellion: A Compilation of the Official Records of the Union and Confederate Armies*. Washington, D.C., 1880–1902. P. 657.

20. M. Lowell. Ibid., 817.

21. Francis L. Black. "Measles Endemicity in Insular Populations: Critical Community Size and Its Evolutionary Implications." *J. Theoret. Biol.* 11 (1966):207.

22. M. S. Bartlett. "Measles Periodicity and Community Size." *J.R. Stat. Soc. Ser.* A120 (1957):40.

23. Rhazes (Al-Razi, Abu Bakr Muhammad). *Med. Class.* 4 (1939):22.

24. T. Sydenham. "The Works of Thomas Sydenham." *Syndenman Soc. (London)* 4 (1922):250.

25. J. F. Anderson and J. Goldberger. "Experimental Measles in the Monkey: A Preliminary Note." *Pub. Health Rep. (Wash.)* 26 (1911):847.

26. Sven Gard. Presentation Speech for the Nobel Award in Physiology and Medicine, 1954.

27. A. Carrel. "Some Conditions of the Reproduction in Vitro of the Rous Virus." *J. Exp. Med.* 43 (1926):647.

28. H. B. Maitland and M. C. Maitland. "Cultivation of Vaccinia Virus." *Lancet* 2 (1928):596.

29. Thomas Weller. "History of Varicella Virus." In *Microbe Hunters Then and Now*, ed. H. Koprowski and M. B. A. Oldstone, pp. 165–72. Bloomington, Ill., 1996.

30. Robert Chanock and Samuel Katz. Personal communication, 1997. Dr. Chanock, a former student of Albert Sabin's, is currently Director of the Laboratory of Infectious Diseases at the National Institutes of Health, Allergy and Infectious Disease Institute, Bethesda, Maryland. Dr. Katz was a student of John Enders's and is currently Professor of Pediatrics at Duke University School of Medicine, Durham, North Carolina.

31. E. Jenner. *A Continuation of Facts and Observations Relative to the Variolae Vaccine, or Cow Pox*. London, 1800.

32. Donald Hopkins. *Princes and Peasants*. Chicago, 1983.

33. F. Home. *Medical Facts and Experiments*. London, 1759.

34. F. Loeffler and P. Frosch. "Berichte der Kommission zur Erforschung der Maul und Klauenseuche bei dem Institut fur Infektionskrankheiten in Berlin." *Zentbl. Bakt. ParasitKde, Abt. I* 23 (1898):371–91.

35. John F. Enders and Thomas C. Peebles. "Propagation in Tissue Culture of Cyto-pathic Agents from Patients with Measles." *Proc. Soc. Exp. Biol. Med.* 86 (1954):277.

36. Editorial, *New York Times*, September 17, 1961.

37. John F. Enders. Letter to the *New York Times*, October 1, 1961.

CHAPTER 7: POLIOMYELITIS

1. Frederick C. Robbins. "Polio—Historical." In *Vaccines*, ed. Stanley Plotkin and Edward Mortimer, Jr., pp. 137–54. Philadelphia, 1994.

2. John R. Paul. *A History of Poliomyelitis.* New Haven, 1971.

3. Sven Gard. Presentation Speech for the Nobel Award in Physiology and Medicine, 1954.

4. Jonas Salk, Jacques A. Drucker, and Denis Malvy. "Non-infectious Poliovirus Vaccine." In *Vaccines*, ed. Plotkin and Mortimer, pp. 205–28.

5. G. Courtois, A. Flack, G. A. Jervis, et al. "Preliminary Report on Mass Vaccination of Man with Live Attenuated Poliomyelitis Virus in the Belgian Congo and Ruanda-Urundi." *Br. Med. J.* 26 (July 1958):187.

6. Hilary Koprowski. "A Visit to Ancient History." In *Microbe Hunters Past and Present*, ed. H. Koprowski and M. B. A. Oldstone, pp. 141–52. Bloomington, Ill., 1996.

7. Albert B. Sabin. "Oral Poliovirus Vaccine: History of Its Development and Use and Current Challenge to Eliminate Poliomyelitis from the World." *J. Infect. Dis.* 151 (1985):420.

8. Thomas Syndenham. "The Works of Thomas Syndenham." *Syndenham Soc. (London)* 2 (1922):250.

9. Michael Underwood. *A Treatise on the Diseases of Children with General Directions for the Management of Infants from the Birth.* London, 1789.

10. Jacob Heine. *Beobach tungen uber Lachmungs zustande der unteren Extremitatien und diren Behandlung.* Stuttgart, 1840.

11. J. M. Charcot. *Lectures on the Diseases of the Nervous System.* London, 1881. Rpt. New York, 1962.

12. Charles Bell. *The Nervous System of the Human Body as Explained in a Series of Papers Read Before the Royal Society of London.* London, 1844.

13. F. Loeffler and P. Frosch. "Berichte der Kommission zur Erforschung der Maul und Klauenseuche bei dem Institut fur Infektionskrankheiten in Berlin." *Zentbl. Bakt. ParasitKde, Abt. I* 23 (1898):371–91.

14. Karl Landsteiner and Edwin Popper. "Mikroscopische Praparate von einem menschlichen und zwei Affenruckenmarken." *Wein. Klin. Wschr.* 21 (1908):1830.

15. Karl Landsteiner and Edwin Popper. "I. Ubertragung der Poliomyelitis Acuta auf Affen." *Z. Immun. Frosch. Exp. Ther.* 2 (1909):377.

16. Karl Landsteiner and Constantin Levaditi. "Surlaparalysie infantile experimente." *C.R. Seanc. Soc. Biol.* 67 (1909):787.

17. Karl Landsteiner and Constantin Levaditi. "La transmission de la paralysie infantile auxsinges." *C.R. Seanc. Soc. Biol.* 67 (1909):592.

18. Simon Flexner and P.A. Lewis. "The Nature of the Virus of Epidemic Poliomyelitis." *J. Am. Med. Assoc.* 53 (1909):2095.

19. *New York Times*, March 9, 1911.

20. Macfarlane Burnet and Jane Macnamara. "Immunologic Differences Between Strains of Poliomyelitic Virus." *Br. J. Exp. Path.* 12 (1931):57.

21. Tony Gould. *A Summer Plague: Polio and Its Survivors.* London, 1995.

22. Al V. Burns. "The Scourge of 1916—America's First and Worst Polio Epidemic." *The American Legion Magazine*, September 1966.

23. *New York Times*, July 7, 1916.

24. *New York Times*, July 14, 1916.

25. Ross T. McIntire. *Twelve Years with Roosevelt.* London, 1948.

26. Geoffrey Ward. *A First Class Temperament: The Emergence of Franklin D. Roosevelt.* New York, 1989.

27. K. Kling, A. Petterson, and W. Wernstedt. *Experimental and Pathological Investigation (Investigations on Epidemic Infantile Paralysis).* State Medical Institute of Sweden, 1912.

28. Joseph L. Melnick. "Enteroviruses: Polioviruses, Coxsackieviruses, Echoviruses, and Newer Enteroviruses." In *Fields' Virology*, ed. B.N. Fields et al., pp. 655–712. New York, 1996.

29. *British Medical Journal*, November 18, 1911.

30. John F. Enders, Frederick C. Robbins, and Thomas H. Weller. "The Cultivation of the Poliomyelitis Viruses in Tissue Culture. Nobel Lecture 1954." *Rev. Infect. Dis.* 2 (1980):493.

31. Joseph L. Melnick. "Live Attenuated Poliovirus Vaccines." In *Vaccines*, ed. Plotkin and Mortimer, pp. 155–204.

32. Richard Carter. *Breakthrough.* New York, 1966.

33. Florian Horaud. "Albert B. Sabin and the Development of Oral Polio Vaccine." *Biologicals* 21 (1993):311.

CHAPTER 8: AN OVERVIEW OF THE HEMORRHAGIC FEVERS

1. Bernard LeGuenno. "Emerging Viruses." *Scientific American*, October 1995.

2. William H. McNeill. *Plagues and Peoples.* New York, 1976.

3. Yves Riviere and Michael B.A. Oldstone. "Genetic Reassortants of Lymphocytic Choriomeningitis Virus: Unexpected Disease and Mechanism of Pathogenesis. *J. Virol.* 59 (1986):363–68.

4. C. Scholtissek, A. Vallbracht, B. Flehmig, and R. Rott. "Correlation of Pathogenicity and Gene Constellation of Influenza A Virus. II. Highly Neurovirulent

Recombinants Derived from Non-Virulent or Weakly Neurovirulent Parent Virus Strains." *Virology* 95 (1979):492–98.

5. D. H. Rubin and B. N. Fields. "Molecular Basis of Reovirus Virulence. Role of the M2 gene." *J. Exp. Med.* 152 (1980):853–57.

6. *Fields' Virology.* Ed. B. N. Fields et al., New York, 1990.

7. M. Salvato, E. Shimomaye, P. Southern, and M. B. A. Oldstone. "Virus-Lymphocyte Interactions. IV. Molecular Characterization of LCMV Armstrong (CTL$^+$) and That of Its Variant, Clone 13 (CTL$^-$)." *Virology* 164 (1988):517–22.

8. M. B. A. Oldstone, M. Salvato, A. Tishon, and H. Lewicki. "Virus-lymphocyte Interactions. III. Biologic Parameters of a Virus Variant That Fails to Generate CTL and Establishes Persistent Infection in Immunocompetent hosts." *Virology* 164 (1988):507–16.

CHAPTER 9: LASSA FEVER

1. Joseph B. McCormick. "Arenaviruses." In *Fields' Virology*, ed. B. N. Fields et al., p. 1245. New York, 1990.

2. John D. Frame, John M. Badwin Jr., David J. Gocke, and Jeanette M. Troup. "Lassa Fever, a New Virus Disease of Man from West Africa." *Am. J. Trop. Med. Hyg.* 19 (1970):670.

3. John D. Frame. "The Story of Lassa Fever. Part I: Discovering the Disease." *N.Y. State J. Med.* 92 (1992):199.

4. John D. Frame. "The Story of Lassa Fever. Part II: Learning More About the Disease." *N.Y. State J. Med.* 92 (1992):264.

5. G. P. Holmes, J. B. McCormick, S. C. Trock, et al. "Lassa Fever in the United States, Investigation of a Case and New Guidelines for Management." *N. Engl. J. Med.* 323 (1990):1120.

CHAPTER 10: EBOLA

1. Frederick A. Murphy, Michael P. Kiley, and Susan P. Fisher-Hoch. "Filoviridae: Marburg and Ebola." In *Fields' Virology*, ed. B. N. Fields et al., p. 933. New York, 1990.

2. B. W. J. Mahy and C. J. Peters. "Current Problems with Viral Hemorrhagic Fevers." In *Microbe Hunters Past and Present*, ed. H. Koprowski and M. B. A. Oldstone, pp. 257–66. Bloomington, Ill., 1996.

3. Bernard LeGuenno. "Emerging Viruses." *Scientific American*, October 1995.

4. *Newsweek*, May 22, 1995.

5. T. W. Geisbert, P. B. Jahrling, M. A. Hanes, et al. "Association of Ebola-Related Reston Virus Particles and Antigen with Tissue Lesions of Monkeys Imported to the United States." *J. Comp. Pathol.* 106 (1992):137.

CHAPTER 11: HANTAVIRUS

1. B. W. J. Mahy and C. J. Peters. "Current Problems with Viral Hemorrhagic Fevers." In *Microbe Hunters Past and Present*, ed. H. Koprowski and M. B. A. Oldstone, pp. 257–66. Bloomington, Ill., 1996.

2. J. M. Hughes, C. J. Peters, M. L. Cohen, and B. W. J. Mahy. "Hantavirus Pulmonary Syndrome: An Emerging Infectious Disease." *Science* 262 (1993):850.

3. L. H. Elliott, T. G. Ksiazek, P. E. Rollin, et al. "Isolation of the Causative Agent of Hantavirus Pulmonary Syndrome." *Am. J. Trop. Med. Hyg.* 51 (1994):102.

4. F. Gonzalez-Scarano and N. Nathanson. "Bunyaviruses." In *Fields' Virology*, ed. B. N. Fields and D. M. Knipe, et al., pp. 1473–1504. New York, 1996.

5. Bernard LeGuenno. "Emerging Viruses." *Scientific American*, October 1995.

CHAPTER 12: HIV—"THE CURRENT PLAGUE"

1. Michael S. Gottlieb, Robert Schroff, Howard M. Schanker, et al. "*Pneumocystis carinii* Pneumonia and Mucosal Candidiasis in Previously Healthy Homosexual Men." *New Engl. J. Med.* 305 (1981):1425.

2. Edward Gelmann, Douglas Blayney, Henry Masur, et al. "Proviral DNA of a Retrovirus, Human T-Cell Leukemia Virus in Two Patients with AIDS." *Science* 220 (1983):862.

3. F. Barré-Sinoussi, J. C. Chermann, F. Rey, et al. "Isolation of a T-Lymphotropic Retrovirus from a Patient at Risk for Acquired Immune Deficiency Syndrome (AIDS)." *Science* 220 (1983):868.

4. Max Essex, M. F. McLane, T. H. Lee, et al. "Antibodies to Cell Membrane Antigens Associated with Human T-Cell Leukemia Virus in Patients with AIDS." *Science* 220 (1983):859.

5. Michael S. Gottlieb, Jerome E. Groopman, Wilfred M. Weinstein, et al. "The Acquired Immunodeficiency Syndrome." *Annals Int. Med.* 99 (1983):208.

6. Martin S. Hirsch and James Curran. "Human Immunodeficiency Viruses." In *Fields' Virology*, ed. B. N. Fields and D. M. Knipe, et al., pp. 1953–76. New York, 1996.

7. Jean Claude Gluckmann. "AIDS Virus History." *Science* 259 (1993):1809.

8. Robert Gallo. *Virus Hunting: AIDS, Cancer and the Human Retrovirus*. New York, 1991.

9. P. Borrow, H. Lewicki, B. H. Hahn, et al. "Virus-Specific CD8$^+$ Cytotoxic T-Lymphocyte Activity Associated with Control of Viremia in Primary Human Immunodeficiency Virus Type 1 Infection." *J. Virol.* 68 (1994):6103.

10. Bruce D. Walker, S. Chakrabati, B. Moss, et al. "HIV Specific Cytotoxic T Lymphocytes in Seropositive Individuals." *Nature* 328 (1987):345.

11. X. Wei, S. K. Ghosh, M. E. Taylor, et al. "Viral Dynamics in Human Immunodeficiency Virus Type 1 Infection." *Science* 373 (1995):117–22.

12. Anthony Fauci. "AIDS: Newer Concepts in the Immunopathogenic Mechanism of Human Immunodeficiency Virus Disease." *Proc. Assoc. Am. Phys.* 107 (1995):1.

13. Clayton Wiley, R. D. Schrier, J. A. Nelson, et al. "Cellular Localization of Human Immunodeficiency Virus Infection Within the Brains of Acquired Immunodeficiency Syndrome Patients." *Proc. Natl. Acad. Sci. USA* 83 (1986):7083.

14. Ashlee V. Moses and Jay A. Nelson. "HIV Infection of Human Brain Capillary Endothelial Cells—Implications for AIDS Dementia." *Adv. Neuroimmunol.* 4 (1994):239–47.

15. F. Loeffler and P. Frosch. "Berichte der Kommission zur Erforschung der Maul und Klauenseuche bei dem Institut Fur Infektionskrankheiten in Berlin." *Zentbl. Bakt. ParasitKde., Abt I* 23 (1898):371–91.

16. V. Ellermann and O. Bang. "Experimentelle Leukamie bei Huhnern." *Zentbl. Bakt. I. Orig.* 46 (1908):595–600.

17. P. Rous. "A Sarcoma of Fowl Transmissible by an Agent Separate from the Tumor Cells." *J. Exp. Med.* 13 (1911):397–411.

18. John B. Moloney. Personal communication.

19. B. J. Poiesz, F. W. Ruscetti, A. F. Gazdar, et al. "Detection and Isolation of Type C Retrovirus Particles from Fresh and Cultured Lymphocytes of a Patient with Cutaneous T-Cell Lymphoma." *Proc. Natl. Acad. Sci. USA* 77 (1980):6815.

20. B. J. Poiesz, F. W. Ruscetti, M. S. Reitz, et al. "Isolation of a New Type C Particle Retrovirus in Primary Uncultured Cells of a Patient with Sezary T-Cell Leukemia." *Nature* 294 (1981):268.

21. D. A. Morgan, F. W. Ruscetti, and R. C. Gallo. "Selective in Vitro Growth of T-Lymphocytes from Normal Human Bone Marrow." *Science* 193 (1976):1007.

22. Y. Hinuma, K. Nagata, M. Hanaoka, et al. "Adult T-Cell Leukemia: Antigen in a CTL Cell Line and Detection of Antibodies to the Antigen in Human Sera." *Proc. Natl. Acad. Sci. USA* 78 (1981):6476.

23. Randy Shilts. *And the Band Played On: Politics, People, and the AIDS Epidemic.* New York, 1987.

24. Jane Kramer. "Bad Blood." *The New Yorker*, October 11, 1993.

CHAPTER 13: SPONGIFORM ENCEPHALOPATHIES

1. C. Besnoit. "La tremblante ou nevrite peripherique enzootique du mouton." *Rev. Vet. Toulouse* 24 (1899):265.

2. J. Cuillé and P. L. Chelle. "Pathologie animal-la maladie dite tremblante du mouton est-elle inoculable." *C.R. Acad. Sci. (Paris)* 203 (1936):1552.

3. J. Cuillé and P. L. Chelle. "Investigations of Scrapie in Sheep." *Vet. Med.* 34 (1939):417.

4. D. C. Gajdusek and V. Zigas. "Degenerative Disease of the Central Nervous System in New Guinea. The Endemic Occurrence of 'Kuru' in the Native Population." *N. Engl. J. Med.* 257 (1957):974.

5. D. C. Gajdusek. "Kuru." *Trans. R. Soc. Trop. Med. Hyg.* 57 (1963):151.

6. D. C. Gajdusek. "Kuru in New Guinea." In *Slow, Latent, and Temperate Virus Infections*, NINDB Monograph No. 2, pp. 3–12. Bethesda, Md., 1965.

7. W. J. Hadlow. "Scrapie and Kuru." *Lancet* 2 (1959):289.

8. B. Chesebro and B. N. Fields. "Transmissible Spongiform Encephalopathies." In *Fields' Virology*, ed. B. N. Fields et al., pp. 2845–50. Philadelphia, 1996.

9. D. C. Gajdusek. "Infectious Amyloids: Subacute Spongiform Encephalopathies as Transmissible Cerebral Amyloidosis." In ibid., 2851–2900.

10. S. B. Prusiner. "Prions." In ibid., 2901–50.

11. R. M. Anderson, C. A. Donnelly, N. M. Ferguson, M. E. J. Woolhouse, C. J. Watt, H. J. Udy, S. MaWhinney, S. P. Dunstan, T. R. E. Southwood, J. W. Wilesmith, J. B. M. Ryan, L. J. Hoinville, J. E. Hillerton, A. R. Austin, and G. A. H. Wells. "Transmission Dynamics and Epidemiology of BSE in British Cattle." *Nature* 382 (1996):779.

12. "BSE Researchers Bemoan Ministry Secrecy." *Nature* 383 (1996):467.

13. D. Butler. "CJD Variant Stirs Debate on Release of Data." *Nature* 384 (1996):658.

14. S. J. Sawyer, G. M. Yuill, T. F. G. Esmore, P. Estibeiro, J. W. Ironside, J. E. Bell, and R. G. Will. "Creutzfeldt-Jakob Disease in an Individual Occupationally Exposed to BSE." *Lancet* 341 (1993):642.

15. P. T. G. Davies, S. Jahfor, I. T. Ferguson, and O. Windi. "Creutzfeldt-Jakob Disease in Individuals Occupationally Exposed to BSE." *Lancet* 342 (1993):680.

16. P. E. M. Smith, M. Ziedler, J. W. Ironside, P. Estibeiro, and T. H. Moss. "Creutzfeldt-Jakob Disease in a Dairy Farmer." *Lancet* 346 (1995):898.

17. T. C. Britton, S. Al-Sarrag, C. Shaw, T. Campbell, and J. Collinge. "Sporadic Creutzfeldt-Jakob Disease in a 16-Year-Old in the UK." *Lancet* 346 (1995):1155.

18. D. Bateman, D. Hilton, S. Love, M. Zeidler, J. Beck, and J. Collinge. "Sporadic Creutzfeldt-Jakob Disease in a 18-Year-Old in the UK." *Lancet* 346 (1995):1155.

19. R. G. Will, J. W. Ironside, M. Ziedler, S. N. Cousens, K. Estibeiro, A. Alperovitch, S. Poser, M. Pocchiari, M. Hofman, and P. G. Smith. "A New Variant of Creutzfeldt-Jakob Disease in the UK." *Lancet* 347 (1996):921.

20. E. Masood. "Mad Cow Scare Threatens Political Link between Food and Agriculture." *Nature* 380 (1996):273.

21. "Lessons from BSE for Public Confidence." *Nature* 380 (1996):271.

22. C. O'Brien. "Scant Data Cause Widespread Concern." *Science* 271 (1996):1798.

23. D. Butler. "Slow Release of Data Adds to BSE Confusion." *Nature* 380 (1996):370.

24. C. Lasmezasi, P. Deslyn, R. Demaimay, K. Adjou, F. Lamoury, D. Dormount, O. Robain, J. Ironside, and J. Hauw. "BSE Transmission to Macaques." *Nature* 381 (1996):743.

25. A. Aguzzi and C. Weissmann. "A Suspicious Signature." *Nature* 383 (1996):666.

26. C. O'Brien. "Protein Test Favors BSE–CJD Link." *Science* 274 (1996):721.

27. J. Collinge, K. Sidle, J. Meads, J. Ironside, and A. Hill. "Molecular Analysis of Prion Strain Variation and the Aetiology of 'New Variant' CJD." *Nature* 383 (1996):685.

28. S. Prusiner. "Novel Proteinaceous Infectious Particles Cause Scrapie." *Science* 216 (1982):136.

29. R. Mestel. "Putting Prions to the Test." *Science* 273 (1996):184.

CHAPTER 14: INFLUENZA VIRUS, THE PLAGUE THAT MAY RETURN

1. Liddell Hart. *A Complete History of the World War*. New York, 1936.

2. Anthony Livesey. *Great Battles of World War I*. New York, 1989.

3. B. Murphy and R. G. Webster. "Orthomyxoviruses." In *Fields' Virology*, ed. B.N. Fields et al., pp. 1397–1446. Philadelphia, 1996.

4. W. Beveridge. *Influenza: The Last Great Plague*. New York, 1978.

5. L. A. Crosby. *Epidemic and Peace, 1918*. Westport Ct.

6. C. H. Stuart-Harris, and G. C. Schild. *Influenza: The Virus and the Disease*. Littleton, Mass., 1976.

7. *Influenza in America 1918–1976*. New York.

8. B. Easterday. "Animal Influenza." In *The Influenza Viruses and Influenza*, ed. E. D. Kilbourne, pp. 449-82. New York, 1975.

9. E. D. Kilbourne. "The Influenza Viruses and Influenza." In *The Influenza Viruses and Influenza*, ed. E. D. Kilbourne. New York, 1975.

10. diCamagliano. *The Chronicles of a Florentine Family, 1200–1470*. 1933.

11. D. O. White, and F. J. Fenner. *Medical Virology*. 1994.

12. T. Willis. "Epidemics in 1658." In *Annals of Influenza*, ed. T. Thompson, p. 11. London, 1885.

13. T. Thompson. *Annals of Influenza or Epidemic Catarrhal Fever in Great Britain from 1510-1837*. London, 1852.

14. Charles Creighton. *A History of Epidemics in Britain*. 1894.

15. Ditmar Finkler. "Influenza." In *Twentieth-Century Practice: An International Encyclopedia of Modern Medical Science by Leading Authorities of Europe and America*, ed. T. L. Stedman, pp. 3-249. New York, 1898.

16. E. S. Thompson. *Influenza*. 1890.

17. J. Skehel. "The Discovery of Human Influenza Virus and Subsequent Influenza Research at the National Institute for Medical Research." In *Microbe Hunters: Then and Now*, ed. H. Koprowski and M. B. A. Oldstone, pp. 205–10. Bloomington, Ill., 1996.

18. J. S. Koen. "A Practical Method for Field Diagnosis of Swine Disease." *Am. J. Vet. Med.* 14 (1919):468.

19. R. E. Shope. "Swine Influenza. I. Experimental Transmission and Pathology." *J. Exp. Med.* 54 (1931):349.

20. R. E. Shope. "Swine Influenza. III. Filtration Experiments and Etiology." *J. Exp. Med.* 54 (1931):373.

21. W. Smith, C. H. Andrews, and P. P. Laidlow. "A Virus Obtained from Influenza Patients." *Lancet* 1 (1933):66.

22. F. M. Burnet. "Influenza Virus on the Developing Egg. I. Changes Associated with the Development of Egg Passaged Strain of Virus." *Br. J. Med. Path.* 17 (1936):282.

23. F. M. Burnet and P. E. Lind. "Studies on Recombination with Influenza Viruses in the Chick Embryo. III. Reciprocal Genetic Interaction Between Two Influenza Virus Strains." *Aust. J. Exp. Med. Sci.* 30 (1952):469.

24. F. M. Burnet. "Influenza Virus Infections of the Chick Embryo by the Amniotic Route." *Aust. J. Exp. Med. Sci.* 18 (1940):353.

25. G. K. Hirst. "The Agglutination of Red Blood Cells by Allantoic Fluid of Chick Embryos Infected with Influenza Virus." *Science* 94 (1941):22.

26. G. K. Hirst. "Adsorption of Influenza Haemagglutinins and Virus by Red Blood Cells." *J. Exp. Med.* 76 (1942):195.

27. R. G. Webster, W. Laver, G. Air, and G. Schild. "Molecular Mechanisms of Variations in Influenza Viruses." *Nature* 296 (1982):115.

28. W. G. Laver and R. G. Webster. "Selection of Antigenic Mutants of Influenza Viruses. Isolation and Peptide Mapping of Their Hemagglutinating Proteins." *Virology* 34 (1968):193.

29. R. G. Webster, C. Campbell, and A. Granoff. "The 'In Vivo' Production of 'New' Influenza A Viruses. I. Genetic Recombination Between Avian and Mammalian Influenza Viruses." *Virology* 44 (971):317.

30. J. K. Taubenberger, A. H. Reid, A. E. Krafft, K. E. Bijwaard, and T. G. Fanning. "Initial Genetic Characterization of the 1918 'Spanish Influenza Virus.'" *Science* 275 (1997):1793–96.

CHAPTER 15: CONCLUSIONS AND FUTURE PREDICTIONS

1. P. de Kruif. *Microbe Hunters.* New York, 1926.

2. P. de Kruif. *The Sweeping Wind.* New York, 1962.

3. World Health Organization. *State of the World's Vaccines and Immunizations.* Geneva, 1996.

AFTERNOTES

1. *New York Times,* 7 March 1999, p. 19.

2. R. G. Will, S. N. Cousens, C. P. Farrington, P. G. Smith, R. S. G. Knight, and J. W. Ironside. "Deaths from Variant Creutzfeldt-Jakob disease." *Lancet* 353 (1999):979; Editorial, "Tragedy of Variant Creutzfeldt-Jakob disease." *Lancet* 353 (1999):939.

3. K. Subbarao, A. Klimov, J. Katz, H. Regnery, W. Lin, H. Hall, M. Perdue, D. Swayne, C. Bender, J. Huang, M. Hemphill, T. Rowe, M. Shaw, X. Xu, K. Fukuda, and N. Cox. "Characterization of an Avian Influenza A (H5N1) Virus Isolated from a Child with Fatal Respiratory Illness." *Science* 279 (1998):393–96.

4. N. Zhou, K. Shortridge, E. Claas, S. Krauss, and R. Webster. "Rapid Evolution of H5N1 Influenza Virus in Chickens in Hong Kong." *J. Virol.* 73 (1999):3366–74.

5. R. Webster, "1918 Spanish Influenza: The Secrets Remain Elusive." *Proc. Natl. Acad. Sci. USA* 96 (1999):1164–66.

6. J. McFarland, L. Baddour, J. Nelson, S. Elkins, R. Craven, B. Croop, G.-J. Chang, A. Grindstaff, A. Craig, and R. Smith. "Imported Yellow Fever in a United States Citizen." *Clin. Infect. Dis.* 25 (1997):1143–47.

7. D.L. Heymann, D. Barakamfitiye, M. Szczeniowski, J.-J. Muyembe-Tamfum, O. Bele, and G. Rodier. "Ebola Hemorrhagic fever: Lessons from Kikwit, Democratic Republic of the Congo." *J. Infect. Dis.* 179:S283–S286.

8. F. Gao, E. Beules, D. Robertson, Y. Chen, C. Rodenburg, S. Michael, L. Cummins, L. Arthur, M. Peeters, G. Shaw, P. Sharp, and B. Hahn. "Origin of HIV-1 in the Chimpanzee *Pantroglodytes Troglodytes*." *Nature* 397 (1999):436–41.

9. Editorial. *Nature* 397 (1999):545.

10. D. Ho. "Too Much Pessimism on AIDS Therapy." *New York Times, O-E,* 27 June 1998.

11. A. Reid, T. Fanning, J. Hultin, and J. Taubenberger. "Origin and Evolution of the 1918 'Spanish' Influenza Virus Hemagglutinin Gene." *Proc. Natl. Acad. Sci. USA* 96 (1999):1651–56.

12. *Nature* 392 (1998):532.

13. N. Bons, N. Mestre-Frances, I. Guiraud, and Y. Charnay. "Prion Immunoreactivity in Brain, Tonsil, Gastrointestinal Epithelial Cells, and Blood and Lymph Vessels in Lemurian Zoo Primates with Spongiform Encephalopathy." *Comptes Rendus de L'Academie des Sciences. Serie III, Sciences de la Vie* 320 (1997):971–79.

14. S. Prusiner. "Prions." *Proc. Natl. Acad. Sci. USA* 95 (1998):13363–83.

15. R. Rhodes. "Pathological Science." *The New Yorker,* 17 December 1997, pp. 54–59.

INDEX